Applied
Body
Composition
Assessment

Vivian H. Heyward, PhD

Lisa M. Stolarczyk, PhD

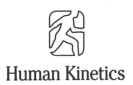

Human Kinetics

Library of Congress Cataloging-in-Publication Data

Heyward, Vivian H.
   Applied body composition assessment / Vivian H. Heyward, Lisa M.
Stolarczyk.
      p. cm.
   Includes bibliographical references and index.
   ISBN 0-87322-653-4 (case text)
   1. Body composition--Measurement.   I. Stolarczyk, Lisa M.
II. Title.
   [DNLM: 1. Body Composition.   2. Anthropometry.   QU 100 H622p
1996]
QP33.5.H49   1996
612--dc20
DNLM/DLC   95-33160
for Library of Congress   CIP

ISBN: 0-87322-653-4

Acquisitions Editor: Richard Washburn; **Developmental Editor:** Elaine Mustain; **Assistant Editors:** Erin Cler, Susan Moore, and John Wentworth; **Editorial Assistants:** Amy Carnes and Andrew Starr; **Copyeditor:** David Frattini; **Proofreader:** Dawn Barker; **Indexer:** Diana Witt; **Typesetter and Text Layout Artist:** Yvonne Winsor; **Text Designer:** Judy Henderson; **Cover Designer:** Keith Blomberg; **Photographer (interior):** Linda K. Gilkey; **Illustrator:** Robert Reuther; **Printer:** Versa Press

Printed in the United States of America   10 9 8 7 6 5 4 3 2 1

Human Kinetics
P.O. Box 5076, Champaign, IL 61825-5076
1-800-747-4457

Canada: Human Kinetics, Box 24040,
Windsor, ON N8Y 4Y9
1-800-465-7301 (in Canada only)

Europe: Human Kinetics,
P.O. Box IW14, Leeds LS16 6TR, United Kingdom
(44) 1132 781708

Australia: Human Kinetics, 2 Ingrid Street,
Clapham 5062, South Australia
(08) 371 3755

New Zealand: Human Kinetics, P.O. Box 105-231, Auckland 1
(09) 523 3462

To all professionals dedicated to improving
the health and physical fitness of their clientele

Acknowledgments

We want to express our appreciation to Timothy Lohman, Fred Newport, and Richard Washburn for their comprehensive reviews of this book. Their comments and suggestions, particularly those on the organization and presentation of material, were extremely beneficial. Special thanks to Rick Frey who made the publication of this book possible and to Elaine Mustain and Erin Cler for their diligent and meticulous work as our developmental and assistant editors. We also would like to acknowledge Brent Ruby and Len Kravitz for their expertise in computer graphics, Linda Gilkey for photography, and Joseph Quatrochi and Kelly Ashbaugh for serving as the models in the photographs.

Contents

How to Use
This Book

As a health or physical fitness professional, you are most likely using body composition field methods, like skinfolds, bioelectrical impedance analysis, near-infrared interactance, and other anthropometric techniques, to measure the body fat of your clients. Like many other practitioners, you may have questions about which body composition method to use. For example, do each of these methods give similar body fat results? Is one method better than the others? If you have a limited budget, which method is most applicable and generalizable to clients differing in age, gender, ethnicity, body fat, and physical activity levels? *Applied Body Composition Assessment* addresses these questions, helps you decide which method to use for certain clients, and tells you how you can refine your techniques and improve your skill as a body composition technician.

Even if you are already using one or more of these body composition methods, you may be confused about which equation to use for each of your clients. For example, can you use the same skinfold equation to measure the body fat of White and Black clients? Elderly and children? Athletes and obese clients? This book not only helps you choose the best method, but enables you to select the best equation based on your client's age, gender, ethnicity, body fat, and physical activity levels. In addition to practical applications, you will find a wealth of theoretical and scientific information that will help you grow professionally by expanding and deepening your understanding of various aspects of body composition.

To use this book you do not need a college degree, or even coursework, in exercise science or an allied health field. However, a basic understanding of human anatomy is beneficial so that you can more easily identify and locate the anatomical landmarks used for skinfold, bioelectrical impedance, near-infrared interactance, and other anthropometric measurements. Also, it is a good idea to read the background information in chapter 1, Body Composition Basics, so you will understand how body composition methods and equations are developed and selected for use, as well as how to use body composition data in your work. If you are presently using a specific method to measure the body fat of your clients, we strongly suggest that you take the time to read the chapter devoted to that method. Detailed information about the skinfold (chapter 2), bioelectrical impedance (chapter 3), near-infrared interactance (chapter 4), and other anthropometric (chapter 5) methods is clearly organized so you can learn about the basic principles of each method, potential sources of measurement error, and how to perfect your technique and skill as a body composition technician.

In the second part of this book, you will find information about measuring body composition of specific population subgroups. Suitable methods and specific equations based on your client's age, gender, ethnicity, body fat, and physical activity level are summarized in tables within each chapter. These equations are also in the Quick Reference Guide at the back of this book (see Appendix A).

To easily identify a suitable method and quickly locate prediction equations for your client in the tables and Quick Reference Guide, you can use the decision trees in Appendix A (see Figures A.1 to A.3). When you are limited to one specific method to measure body fat, you can use the equation finders developed for the skinfold, bioelectrical impedance, near-infrared interactance, and other anthropometric methods (see Appendix A: Figures A.4a to A.7). As you work your way through the decision tree or equation finder, an equation suitable for your client is identified. You can find this equation by looking for the equation number in either the text (see table and page number) or Quick Reference Guide (see Appendix A and page number).

Although using selected equations for specific population subgroups will give a more accurate assessment of your client's body composition, a major drawback is the time it takes to identify the prediction equation and to do the calculations for each client. To handle this problem, complementary computer software by Nelson Ng is available from Human Kinetics. With this software, you will be able to quickly identify suitable methods and equations for your clients.

It is our hope that this book increases your understanding and appreciation for both the art and science of body composition assessment, further develops your knowledge and skill as a body composition technician, and helps you provide your clients with the most accurate information about their body composition.

Part I

Body Composition Methodology

Chapter 1

Body Composition Basics

Obesity is a serious health problem that reduces life expectancy by increasing one's risk of developing coronary artery disease, hypertension, Type II diabetes, obstructive pulmonary disease, osteoarthritis, and certain types of cancer. The prevalence of hypertension, hyperlipidemia, and Type II diabetes is two to three times greater in obese individuals (National Institutes of Health [NIH], 1985). According to the most recent National Health and Nutrition Examination Survey (NHANES III), 58 million, or one out of every three (33%), adults in the United States are overweight (Kuczmarski, Flegal, Campbell, & Johnson, 1994). The increased health risks associated with obesity are related, not only to the total amount of body fat, but also to the way in which fat is distributed, especially in the abdominal region (intra-abdominal or visceral fat). Visceral fat is a stronger predictor of cardiovascular disease and other metabolic disorders, such as Type II diabetes, than overall body fat (Bjorntorp, 1985, 1990).

Too little body fat, however, also poses a health risk because the body needs a certain amount of fat for normal physiological functions. Essential lipids, like phospholipids, are needed for cell membrane formation, while nonessential lipids, like triglycerides found in adipose tissue, provide thermal insulation and store metabolic fuel (free-fatty acids). In addition, lipids are involved in the transport and storage of fat-soluble vitamins (A, D, E, and K), in the functioning of the nervous system, the menstrual cycle, and the reproductive system, as well as growth and maturation during pubescence. Thus, too little body fatness, as found in individuals with eating disorders (anorexia nervosa), exercise addiction, and certain diseases such as cystic fibrosis, can lead to serious physiological dysfunction. Because of the health risks associated with abnormal amounts of body fat on either end of the scale, health professionals need to understand the principles underlying the assessment of total body composition and regional fat distribution.

In the NHANES III (Kuczmarski et al., 1994), overweight is defined as a body mass index (weight/height squared) greater than or equal to 27.8 kg/m^2 for men and 27.3 kg/m^2 for women, which represents approximately 124% of desirable body weight for men and 120% of desirable weight for women. This definition is inadequate because it does not take into account the body composition of the individual. Use of height and weight tables enforces the misconception that body weight is more important than body fatness. Many people are concerned about losing body weight and being thin, without recognizing that there is an important distinction between being thin and being lean. While thinness is related to body weight, leanness is associated with the composition of the individual's body weight. Thin individuals may weigh less than the recommended value in height-weight tables, whereas lean individuals with little body fat may weigh more than their ideal, tabled body weight because of increased muscle and bone mass (i.e., muscle and bone weigh more than fat). Similarly, some individuals may be overfat or obese even though they are not overweight. Thus, using height-weight norms can lead to an erroneous conclusion about one's level of body fatness and health risk. *Obesity is better defined as an excessive amount of total body fat for a given body weight.*

The amount of body fat is quantified by assessing the fat mass (FM) and fat-free mass (FFM) of the individual. The FM includes all extractable lipids from adipose and other tissues. The FFM consists of all residual chemicals and tissues, including water, muscle, bone, connective tissues, and internal organs. Although the terms FFM and lean body mass (LBM) are sometimes used interchangeably, there is a distinction. Unlike FFM, which contains no lipids, the LBM includes a small amount (2% to 3% in males and 5% to 8% in females) of essential lipids (Lohman, 1992). Table 1.1 defines some terms commonly used in the body composition field. For a more extensive list of definitions, refer to the glossary beginning on page 190.

To classify level of body fatness, the relative body fat (%BF) is obtained by dividing the FM by the total body weight (BW): %BF = (FM/BW) × 100. The estimates for body fatness, as recommended by Lohman (1992), are presented in Table 1.2. The average %BF is 15 for men and 23 for women. The standard for obesity that places an individual at risk for disease is body fat in excess of 25% for men and 32% for women. Minimum healthy fat levels are estimated to be 5% for men and 8% to 12% for women.

Table 1.1   Body Composition Terminology

Terminology	Definition
Fat mass (FM)	All extractable lipids from adipose and other tissues in the body.
Adipose tissue mass (ATM)	Fat (~83%) plus its supporting structures (~2% protein and ~15% water).
Fat-free mass (FFM) or fat-free body (FFB)	All residual, lipid-free chemicals and tissues, including water, muscle, bone connective tissue and internal organs.
Lean body mass (LBM)	FFM plus essential lipids.
Relative body fat (%BF)	FM expressed as a percentage of total body weight.
Essential lipids	Compound lipids (phospholipids) needed for cell membrane formation ~10% of total-body lipid.
Nonessential lipids	Triglycerides found primarily in adipose tissue ~90% of total body lipid.
Total body density (Db)	Total body mass expressed relative to total body volume.
Subcutaneous fat	Adipose tissue stored underneath the skin.
Visceral fat	Adipose tissue within and around the organs in the thoracic (e.g., heart, lungs) and abdominal (e.g., liver, kidneys) cavities.
Intra-abdominal fat	Visceral fat in the abdominal cavity.
Abdominal fat	Subcutaneous and visceral fat in the abdominal region.

Body Composition Field Methods

Anthropometry has been used for over a century to assess body size and the proportions of body segments by measuring body circumferences and body segments. As early as 1915, the thickness of subcutaneous adipose tissue was measured by taking skinfold (SKF) measurements. Later, in the 1960s and 1970s, these measures were used to develop numerous anthropometric equations for predicting the total body density (Db) and body fat. At present, there are excellent anthropometric equations that use either SKF or circumferences and diameters to estimate body composition. These tests are suitable for field and clinical settings because they are easy to administer to large groups at a relatively low cost; the price of anthropometric tape

Table 1.2   Percent Body Fat Standards for Men and Women

	Men	Women
At risk[a]	≤5%	≤8%
Below average	6–14%	9–22%
Average	15%	23%
Above average	16–24%	24–31%
At risk[b]	≥25%	≥32%

Note. Data from Lohman (1992, p. 80).

[a]At risk for diseases and disorders associated with malnutrition

[b]At risk for diseases associated with obesity

measures and SKF calipers range from $10 to $350. However, the accuracy of the SKF method is affected by the skill of the SKF technician. The technician who is not properly trained will introduce significant measurement error, which leads to an inaccurate estimate of the client's body composition.

Another body composition method suitable to field and clinical settings is bioelectrical impedance analysis (BIA). This technique was pioneered in the early 1960s, and since that time, equations have been developed, based on age, gender, level of body fatness, race, and physical activity level, to accurately estimate the FFM and body fat of various groups.

BIA is rapid and noninvasive but more expensive than SKF and anthropometric methods (the cost of BIA analyzers ranges from $3,000 to $4,500). However, compared to the SKF and anthropometric techniques, this method does not require as much training and practice to become a skilled technician. A major limitation of BIA is that your clients must adhere to strict pretest guidelines in order to yield valid estimates of their body composition.

In the late 1980s, a new field method, near-infrared interactance (NIR), was developed and marketed for body composition assessment. This method is rapid, safe, and uses a low-cost ($2,000) near-infrared analyzer to estimate %BF. However, compared to SKF and BIA, which have been validated and refined through years of research, NIR is still in developmental stages. To date there is much skepticism surrounding the use of NIR to assess body composition.

Body Composition Applications

In addition to assessing total body fat and regional body fat to identify your clients' health risks, there are other important ways that body composition measures can be used by medical, health, and fitness professionals (Table 1.3).

Table 1.3   Body Composition Applications

- To identify the client's health risk associated with excessively low or high levels of total body fat
- To identify the client's health risk associated with excessive accumulation of intra-abdominal fat
- To promote the client's understanding of health risks associated with too little or too much body fat
- To monitor changes in body composition that are associated with certain diseases
- To assess the effectiveness of nutrition and exercise interventions in altering body composition
- To estimate ideal body weight of clients and athletes
- To formulate dietary recommendations and exercise prescriptions
- To monitor growth, development, maturation, and age-related changes in body composition

Monitoring changes in FFM and FM can further our understanding of energy metabolism and of various diseases that alter body composition. This understanding could lead to the development of more effective nutrition and exercise intervention strategies to counteract the loss of FFM associated with factors such as malnutrition, aging, injury, and certain diseases. Body composition is often assessed in patients with AIDS (Rabeneck, Risser, Crane, McCabe, & Worsley, 1993), anorexia nervosa (Mazess, Barden, & Ohlrich, 1990), cancer (Fredrix et al., 1990), chronic obstructive pulmonary disease (Schols, Wouters, Soeters, & Westerterp, 1991), cirrhosis (Zillikens, van den Berg, Wilson, Rietveld, & Swart, 1992), coronary heart disease (Tanaka et al., 1993), cystic fibrosis (Spicher, Roulet, Schaffner, & Schultz, 1993), end-stage renal disease and renal transplants (Hart, Wilkie, Edwards, & Cunningham, 1993; Saxenhofer, Scheidegger, Descoeudres, Jaeger, & Horber, 1992), heart transplants (Keteyian et al., 1992), and spinal cord injuries (George, Wells, & Dugan, 1988).

Another important facet of body composition is the estimation of a healthy body weight and the formulation of dietary recommendations and exercise prescriptions, especially for obese individuals. Too often, obesity and weight management clinics focus on total-body weight loss rather than fat loss. The most effective way of creating a caloric deficit to maximize fat loss is through a combination of diet (reduced caloric intake) and exercise (aerobics and weight training). A high carbohydrate-low fat diet can prevent the depletion of muscle glycogen stores and maximize the protein-sparing effect of carbohydrates to help preserve FFM. Weight training also counteracts the loss of FFM associated with caloric restriction by increasing muscle and bone mass.

Additionally, low-to-moderate intensity aerobic exercise increases fat mobilization and utilization for energy production and is an effective way of reducing body fat (Pavlou, Steffee, Lerman, & Burrows, 1985).

Accurate assessment of a healthy body weight is also important for athletes in sports, such as wrestling, power-lifting, and bodybuilding, that use body weight classifications for competition. Many of these athletes use acute weight loss techniques (e.g., saunas, fluid deprivation, diuretics, and fasting) in order to dehydrate the body and reach a specific body weight for competition. Although the American Medical Association (1967) and the American College of Sports Medicine (1985) have issued position statements and guidelines regarding weight control for wrestlers, the unsafe practices associated with "making weight" continue to be used (Steen & Brownell, 1990).

The problems associated with achieving a healthy body weight and body composition for optimal physical performance are not confined either to sports using weight classification for competition or to male athletes. Recently, the American College of Sports Medicine (1992) produced a slide presentation to inform coaches, physical educators, and athletic trainers about the prevalence, detection, and treatment of eating disorders among female athletes. Although methods are available for accurately estimating a healthy body weight and body composition for athletes in different sports (see chapter 10), coaches and athletic trainers have not used them very much to ensure the health and well-being of their athletes.

Finally, physical educators and parents can use body composition measures both to monitor children's growth and to identify those at risk because of over- or underfatness. Lohman (1992) reported that the prevalence of obesity in boys and girls, 6 to 11 years old, increased 62% and 65%, respectively, between 1960 and 1980. Williams, Going, Lohman, Harsha, et al. (1992) demonstrated that the %BF (estimated from SKF) of boys and girls, ages 5 to 18 years, was linked to coronary heart disease risk factors (blood pressure, total cholesterol, and lipoprotein ratios) in children and adolescents. In addition, many children have inaccurate perceptions of their body fatness and distorted body images, contributing to the high rate of eating disorders for middle school and high school students (Slavin, 1988). Body composition assessment, as well as information concerning healthy levels of body fatness, needs to be incorporated into health and physical education curricula.

Body Composition Models

Theoretical models are used to obtain reference measures of body composition for the development of anthropometric, skinfold, bioelectrical impedance, and near-infrared interactance methods and equations. To study body composition, the body weight is subdivided into two or more compartments using elemental, chemical, anatomic, or fluid-metabolic models (Figure 1.1). Generally, the chemical and whole-body models have been more widely used in body composition research. The classic two-component model divides the body mass into fat and fat-free body (FFB) compartments. The fat consists of all extractable lipids, and the FFB includes water, protein, and mineral components (Siri, 1961). The densities of fat (0.901 grams per cubic centimeter or g/cc) and FFB (1.10 g/cc) for a "reference body" were based on measurements observed from dissection of only three white male cadavers, 25, 35, and 46 years of age (Brozek, Grande, Anderson, & Keys, 1963). The FFB density was calculated using the relative proportions and corresponding densities of each FFB component of these cadavers (Table 1.4).

Applying this two-component model requires the following assumptions (Brozek et al., 1963; Siri, 1961):

1. The density of fat is 0.901 g/cc.
2. The density of the FFB is 1.10 g/cc.
3. The densities of fat and the FFB components (water, protein, mineral) are the same for all individuals.
4. The densities of the tissues comprising the FFB are constant within an individual, and their porportional contribution to the lean component remains constant.
5. The individual being measured differs from the reference body only in the amount of fat. The FFB of the reference body is assumed to be 73.8% water, 19.4% protein, and 6.8% mineral.

This two-component model has served as the cornerstone upon which the hydrodensitometry (underwater weighing) method is based. Using the assumed proportions and their respective densities (Table 1.4), equations can be derived to convert the individual's total body density (Db) from hydrostatic weighing into relative body fat proportions (%BF). Two commonly used equations are the Siri (1961) equation, %BF = [(4.95/Db) − 4.50] × 100, and the Brozek et al. (1963) equation, %BF = [(4.57/Db) − 4.142] × 100. These

Table 1.4   Assumed Values for Fat and Fat-Free Body (FFB) Components

Component	Density (g/cc)	Proportion (%)
Fat	0.9007	15.3
FFB	1.1000	84.7
Water	*0.9937*	*73.8*
Protein	*1.34*	*19.4*
Mineral	*3.038*	*6.8*

Note. Data from Brozek et al. (1963, pp. 123-124).

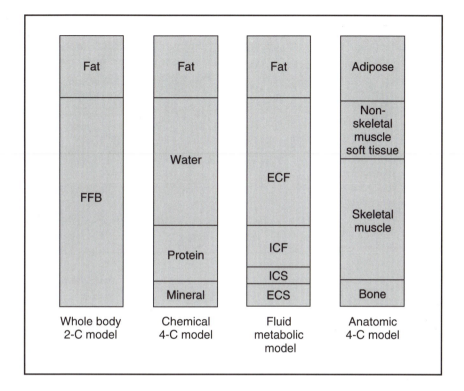

Figure 1.1 Two-component (2-C) and multicomponent body composition models. ECF = extracellular fluid; ICF = intracellular fluid; ICS = intracellular solids; ECS = extracellular solids.

two equations yield similar %BF estimates for body densities ranging from 1.0300 to 1.0900 g/cc. For example, if a client's measured body density is 1.0500 g/cc, the %BF estimates, obtained by plugging this value into the Siri and Brozek et al. equations, are 21.4% and 21.0%, respectively.

Generally, two-component model equations provide accurate estimates of %BF as long as the basic assumptions of the model are met. However, there is no guarantee that the FFB composition of an individual within a certain population subgroup will exactly match the values assumed for the reference body. In fact, researchers have reported that these equations produce systematic prediction error when they are applied to population subgroups whose FFB density varies from the assumed value (1.10 g/cc) used to derive these equations.

Recent technological advances for measuring the water (isotope dilution), mineral (dual-energy x-ray absorptiometry), and protein (neutron activation analysis) compartments of the FFB have allowed researchers to quantify the

Table 1.5 Estimations of FFB Density Derived From Multicomponent Models for Population Subgroups

	Subgroup	FFB$_d$[a] (g/cc)	Range	Reference
Males				
White	Prepubescent (7-12 yr)	1.084	NR	Lohman (1986)
	Pubescent (13-16 yr)	1.094	NR	Lohman (1986)
	Postpubescent (17-19 yr)	1.098	NR	Lohman (1986)
	Adult (19-24 yr)	1.103	1.096-1.110	Friedl et al. (1992)
	Adult (18-55 yr)	1.102	1.080-1.111	Fuller et al. (1992)
	Adult (22-75 yr)	1.102	1.082-1.122	Clark, Kuta, & Sullivan (1993)
	Adult (42-94 yr)	1.094	1.082-1.104	Heymsfield et al. (1989)
Black	Adult (18-32 yr)	1.113	NR	Schutte et al. (1984)
Females				
White	Prepubescent (7-12 yr)	1.082	NR	Lohman (1986)
	Pubescent (13-16 yr)	1.093	NR	Lohman (1986)
	Postpubescent (17-19 yr)	1.095	NR	Lohman (1986)
	Adult (24-78 yr)	1.097	1.070-1.114	Ortiz et al. (1992)
	Adult (24-85 yr)	1.097	1.087-1.103	Heymsfield et al. (1989)
	Adult (20-59 yr)	1.100	1.080-1.111	Fuller et al. (1992)
Black	Adult (24-79 yr)	1.106	1.091-1.146	Ortiz (1992)
Hispanic	Adult (20-40 yr)	1.105	NR	Stolarczyk et al. (1995)
American Indian	Adult (18-60 yr)	1.108	NR	Hicks (1992)

NR = not reported

[a]Fat-free body density

FFB composition in vivo using multicomponent models that take into account individual variation in the water and mineral compartments of the FFB. These studies (Table 1.5) demonstrate surprisingly good agreement between the assumed FFB density (1.10 g/cc) and the multicomponent model estimates (1.102 to 1.103 g/cc) for white males, 19 to 55 years of age (Friedl, DeLuca, Marchitelli, & Vogel, 1992; Fuller, Jebb, Laskey, Coward, & Elia, 1992), indicating that the Siri and Brozek et al. equations can be used to accurately estimate %BF in white males.

Other researchers have reported that FFB density varies with age, gender, ethnicity, level of body fatness, and physical activity level, depending mainly on the relative proportion of water and mineral comprising the FFB (Baum-gartner, Heymsfield, Lichtman, Wang, & Pierson, 1991; Wang, Heymsfield, Aulet, Thornton, & Pierson, 1989; Williams et al., 1993). For example, the FFB densities of black women (1.106 g/cc) and black men (1.113 g/cc) are greater than 1.10 g/cc because of their higher mineral content (~7.3% FFB) and bone density (Deck-Cote & Adams, 1993; Ortiz et al., 1992; Schutte et al., 1984). Because of this difference in FFB density, the body fat of blacks will be systematically underestimated when two-component model equations are used to estimate %BF. Likewise, the FFB density of children is estimated to be only 1.084 g/cc because of their relative lower mineral (5.2% FFB) and higher body water (76.6% FFB) compared to the reference body (Lohman, Boileau, & Slaughter, 1984). Also, the average density of the FFB of elderly men and women is 1.096 g/cc because of the relatively low body mineral value (6.2% FFB) in this population (Heymsfield et al., 1989). Thus, the relative body fat of children and the elderly will be systematically overesti-mated using two-component model equations.

Although the average FFB density for certain population subgroups (Table 1.5) may be very close to the assumed value (1.10 g/cc), it is important to note the high degree of interindividual variation within any given subpopu-lation. For this reason, there is a need to use body composition prediction equations that are validated against a reference body composition measure derived from multicomponent models. It is unfortunate that the overwhelm-ing majority of existing field methods and prediction equations were devel-oped using hydrodensitometry and two-component model equations to derive reference measures of %BF and FFM. However, there are some SKF and BIA equations that were developed using multicomponent model refer-ence measures (Boileau, Lohman, & Slaughter, 1985; Horswill, Lohman, Slaughter, Boileau, & Wilmore, 1990; Lohman, 1986, 1992; Slaughter et al., 1988; Stolarczyk, Heyward, Hicks, & Baumgartner, 1994). Alternatively, some SKF, BIA, and NIR equations estimate Db instead of %BF or FFM. For these equations, the estimated Db can be converted to %BF by using conversion formulas derived for specific population subgroups. These popu-lation-specific conversion formulas (Table 1.6) were calculated using multi-component model estimates of FFB density obtained from the literature (see the footnotes to Table 1.6 for specific references).

Selecting Valid Field Methods and Equations

As a body composition practitioner, you need to be able to evaluate the relative worth of body composition field methods and equations. This is especially true given that researchers are presently developing new SKF, BIA, and NIR equations using multicomponent models to obtain reference measures of body composition. To develop body composition prediction

Table 1.6 Population-Specific Formulas for Conversion of Db to %BF

Population	Age	Gender	%BF	FFB_d (g/cc)
Race				
American Indian	18-60	Female	(4.81/Db) − 4.34	1.108[a]
Black	18-32	Male	(4.37/Db) − 3.93	1.113
	24-79	Female	(4.85/Db) − 4.39	1.106[b]
Hispanic	20-40	Female	(4.87/Db) − 4.41	1.105[c]
Japanese Native	18-48	Male	(4.97/Db) − 4.52	1.099[d]
		Female	(4.76/Db) − 4.28	1.111[e]
	61-78	Male	(4.87/Db) − 4.41	1.105[f]
		Female	(4.95/Db) − 4.50	1.100[g]
White	7-12	Male	(5.30/Db) − 4.89	1.084
		Female	(5.35/Db) − 4.95	1.082
	13-16	Male	(5.07/Db) − 4.64	1.094
		Female	(5.10/Db) − 4.66	1.093
	17-19	Male	(4.99/Db) − 4.55	1.098
		Female	(5.05/Db) − 4.62	1.095
	20-80	Male	(4.95/Db) − 4.50	1.100
		Female	(5.01/Db) − 4.57	1.097
Levels of body fatness				
Anorexic	15-30	Female	(5.26/Db) − 4.83	1.087[h]
Obese	17-62	Female	(5.00/Db) − 4.56	1.098[i]

[a]Assumes water and protein proportions are 73% and 18.9%, respectively. Measured mineral was 8.1% FFB (Hicks, 1992).

[b]Assumes protein proportion is 19.2%. Measured mineral was 7.8% FFB and water was 73% FFB (Ortiz et al., 1992).

[c]Assumes protein proportion is 19.8%. Measured mineral was 7.4% FFB and water was 72.8% FFB (Stolarczyk et al., 1995).

[d]Assumes water and protein proportions are 73% and 20.7%, respectively. Measured mineral was 6.3% FFB (Tsunenari et al., 1993).

[e]Assumes water and protein proportions are 73% and 18.4%, respectively. Measured mineral was 8.6% FFB (Tsunenari et al., 1993).

[f]Assumes water and protein proportions are 73% and 19.6%, respectively. Measured mineral was 7.4% FFB (Tsunenari et al., 1993).

[g]Assumes water and protein proportions are 73% and 20.4%, respectively. Measured mineral was 6.6% FFB (Tsunenari et al., 1993).

[h]Assumes protein proportion is 17.7%. Measured water and mineral were 76% and 6.3% FFB, respectively. Mineral density was estimated at 2.73 g/cc (Dempsey et al., 1984; Mazess, Barden, & Ohlrich, 1990).

[i]Assumes protein proportion is 16%. Measured water and mineral were 76% and 8% FFB, respectively (Albu et al., 1989; Lindsay et al., 1992; Segal, Wang, et al., 1987).

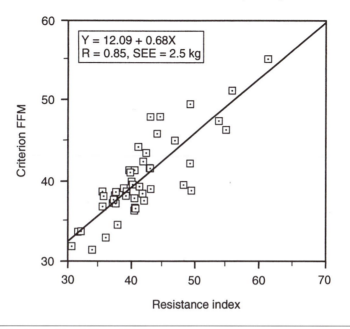

Figure 1.2 Line of best fit and SEE.

equations, researchers commonly use a statistical technique called multiple regression. This technique allows researchers to identify an equation that uses the best combination of measured variables for predicting the reference body composition measure, such as Db or FFM. For example, a skinfold prediction equation may include the sum of three skinfolds and the individual's age to estimate Db.

Good prediction equations yield a high correlation (termed the multiple correlation coefficient or R_{mc}) between the reference measure (what is being predicted) and the combination of measured variables used to predict it (predictor variables). The value of the reference measure is estimated with a small degree of error (standard error of estimate or SEE), meaning that the individual's predicted score is close in value to that individual's reference measure. The relationship between the reference measure and the predictors is best illustrated in a scatterplot (Figure 1.2). The line fitted through the data points is the line of best fit (regression line). When the standard error of estimate is small, the data points do not deviate much from the line of best fit. In fact, if an equation predicted each individual's reference score perfectly, all data points would fall along the line of best fit.

To use the prediction equation, the individual's score for each predictor variable is multiplied by its respective constant value. All of the products are added together to yield a predicted score for the individual. The constants (regression weights) for the predictor variables are obtained from the multiple regression analysis. A good prediction equation has stable regression

Table 1.7   Multicomponent Model Equations

	Reference
Three-Component	
%BF = [(2.118/Db) − 0.78W − 1.354] × 100	Siri (1961)
%BF = [(6.386/Db) + 3.961M − 6.090] × 100	Lohman (1986)
Four-Component	
%BF = [(2.559/Db) − 0.734W + 0.983M − 1.841] × 100	Friedl et al. (1992)
%BF = [(2.747/Db) − 0.714W + 1.146B − 2.053] × 100	Selinger (1977)

BW = body weight (kg)

W = TBW (l)/BW (kg)

M = TBM (kg)/BW (kg)

B = osseous mineral (kg)/BW (kg)

weights, meaning that their values do not change much from group to group. To obtain stable regression weights, the researcher must use a large number of subjects (100 to 400) when developing the prediction equation. The stability of the regression weights for each predictor in the equation is tested by applying the prediction equation to another sample of subjects (the cross-validation sample) and comparing these regression weights to those derived for the original sample (the validation sample). To further establish the applicability of the prediction equation to other independent samples from the population, additional cross-validation procedures are performed (see steps 6-9, pp. 18-19).

To select the most appropriate equations to use for your clients, it is important to evaluate the relative worth of the body composition field methods and prediction equations. You should ask the following questions:

1. *What body composition reference method was used to develop this equation?* Many experts in the body composition field view hydrodensitometry as the best method for measuring body composition, provided that

  a. appropriate, population-specific conversion formulas are used to convert Db to %BF, or
  b. multicomponent model equations, adjusted for individual variation in relative total body water (TBW) and/or total body mineral (TBM), are used to estimate %BF from Db.

Some of these multicomponent model equations for estimating reference %BF from hydrodensitometry are listed in Table 1.7. In addition, to ensure the precision and accuracy of hydrodensitometry, the individual's residual lung volume (RV), or the volume of air left in the lung after a maximal expiration, must be measured directly (helium-, nitrogen-, or oxygen-dilution methods) and must not be predicted from RV equations. Using a predicted RV produces large measurement errors (2.8 %BF to 3.7 %BF) that are unacceptable (Morrow, Jackson, Bradley, & Hartung, 1986).

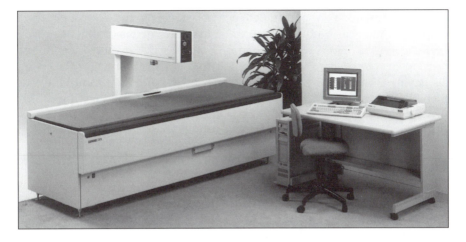

Figure 1.3   Dual-energy x-ray absorptiometer.

Dual-energy x-ray absorptiometry (DXA) is a relatively new technology that is gaining recognition as a reference method for body composition research (Figure 1.3). This method yields estimates of bone mineral, fat, and lean soft-tissue mass. DXA is highly reliable (Mazess, Barden, Bisek, & Hanson, 1990), and there is good agreement between %BF estimates obtained by hydrodensitometry and by DXA (Going et al., 1993; Hicks, Heyward, Baumgartner, et al., 1993; Van Loan & Mayclin, 1992). DXA is an attractive alternative to hydrodensitometry as a reference method because it is safe, rapid (a total body scan takes 10 to 20 minutes), requires minimal subject cooperation, and most importantly, accounts for individual variability in bone mineral. In the future, it is highly likely that body composition prediction equations will be developed and validated using DXA as a reference method. However, further research is needed before DXA can be firmly established as the best reference method (Roubenoff, Kehayias, Dawson-Hughes, & Heymsfield, 1993). It is important to note that the DXA method has not yet been approved by the Food and Drug Administration of the United States. Therefore, you will need Institutional Review Board approval when using this method in research and clinical settings.

The reference measure estimated from the prediction equation varies depending on the field method. Typically, SKF and NIR equations predict either Db or %BF. The individual skinfolds and the sum of skinfolds from multiple sites are inversely related to Db. In other words, the greater the sum of skinfolds, the lower the body density, indicating a greater %BF for the individual. Likewise, the optical density (OD) at the biceps site (measured by NIR) is inversely related to %BF. The higher the OD value, the lower the %BF.

BIA equations generally predict the individual's TBW or FFM, rather than Db or %BF, because of the theoretically derived relationship between the volume of TBW or FFM and impedance (resistance) to the flow of electrical current through the body. Because water and electrolytes conduct electrical current, and the FFM is comprised mostly of water (73%), there is an inverse relationship between impedance and TBW or FFM. In other words, individuals having a large FFM will have a smaller impedance to current flow. The theoretical principles and assumptions for each of these field methods (SKF, BIA, and NIR) are explained in greater detail in chapters 2, 3, and 4, respectively.

2. *How large was the sample used to develop the prediction equation? What is the ratio of sample size to the number of predictor variables in the equation?* Generally, large, randomly-selected samples (N = 100 to 400 subjects) are needed to ensure that the data are representative of the population for whom the equation was developed. Equations based on large samples tend to have more stable regression weights for each predictor variable in the equation. In multiple regression, the correlation between the reference body composition variable (Db, %BF, or FFM) and the predictors in the equation is represented by the multiple correlation coefficient (R_{mc}). The larger the R_{mc} (to a maximum value of 1.00), the stronger the relationship. The size of R_{mc} will be artificially inflated if there are too many predictors in the equation compared to the total number of subjects. Statisticians recommend that there should be a minimum of 10 to 20 subjects per predictor variable (Pedhazuer, 1982). For example, if a SKF prediction equation has three predictors (e.g., triceps SKF, calf SKF, and age), then the minimum sample size needs to be 30 to 60 subjects. Prediction equations that are based on small samples and have a poor subject-to-predictor ratio are suspect and should not be used.

3. *What was the size of the R_{mc} and the standard error of estimate (SEE) for this equation?* In general, the R_{mc} for body composition prediction equations exceeds 0.80. This means that at least 64%, [$R^2 = (0.80)^2 \times 100$] of variance in the reference measure can be accounted for by the predictors in the equation. As you can easily see, the larger the R_{mc}, the greater the amount of shared variance between the reference measure and predictors. When you evaluate the relative worth of a prediction equation, it is more important to note the size of the SEE instead of the R_{mc} because the magnitude of R_{mc} is greatly affected by the size and variability of the sample.

The SEE reflects the degree of deviation of individual data points (subject's scores) around the line of best fit through the entire sample's data points. The line of best fit is the regression line which depicts the linear relationship between the reference measure and the predictors. The closer individual data points fall near the regression line, the smaller the SEE or prediction error (Figure 1.2). Lohman (1992) developed standards for evaluating prediction errors of body composition equations estimating %BF and FFM. These values are based on empirically derived measurement errors associated with

Table 1.8   Standards for Evaluating Prediction Errors (SEE)

SEE %BF male and female	SEE Db (g/cc) male and female	SEE FFM (kg) male	SEE FFM (kg) female	Subjective rating
2.0	0.0045	2.0-2.5	1.5-1.8	Ideal
2.5	0.0055	2.5	1.8	Excellent
3.0	0.0070	3.0	2.3	Very good
3.5	0.0080	3.5	2.8	Good
4.0	0.0090	4.0	2.8	Fairly good
4.5	0.0100	4.5	3.6	Fair
5.0	0.0110	> 4.5	> 4.0	Poor

Note. Data from Lohman (1992, pp. 3-4).

the reference method (hydrodensitometry). Standards for evaluating the SEE for %BF, Db, and FFM are presented in Table 1.8.

4. *To whom is the prediction equation applicable?* To answer this question, you need to pay close attention to the physical characteristics of the sample used to derive the equation. Factors such as age, gender, race, level of body fatness, and physical activity level need to be examined carefully. Prediction equations are either population-specific or generalized. Population-specific equations are intended to be used only to estimate the body composition of individuals from a specific homogeneous group. For example, there are separate SKF equations developed for prepubescent black males and prepubescent white males (Slaughter et al., 1988). Population-specific equations are likely to systematically over- or underestimate body composition if they are applied to individuals who do not belong to that population subgroup.

There are generalized prediction equations that can be applied to individuals who differ greatly in physical characteristics. Generalized equations are developed using diverse, heterogeneous samples and account for differences in physical characteristics by including these variables as predictors in the equation. For example, the generalized BIA equation of Van Loan and Mayclin (1987) can be applied to both men and women, ranging in age from 18 to 60 years, because gender and age are predictors in this equation. Likewise, age is a predictor in the Jackson, Pollock, and Ward (1980) SKF equation. Therefore, this equation is generalizable to women from 18 to 55 years of age. In later chapters, population-specific and generalized body composition prediction equations are presented for various ages (children and the elderly), races (American Indians, blacks, Hispanics, Japanese Natives, and whites), levels of fatness (anorexics and obese), and physical activity levels (athletes).

5. *How were the variables measured by the researchers who developed the prediction equation?* It is not only important to know which variables are included in a prediction equation, but also how each one of these predictors was measured by the researchers developing the equation. Although it is highly recommended that standardized anthropometric procedures and measurement sites be used in all body composition studies, this is not always the case. For example, the suprailiac skinfold used in the skinfold equations developed by Jackson et al. (1980) is measured above the iliac crest at the anterior axillary line. In contrast, Lohman, Roche, and Martorell (1988) recommend that the suprailiac skinfold be measured above the iliac crest at the midaxillary line. For most individuals, there will be a difference between skinfold thicknesses measured at these two sites. Thus, larger-than-expected prediction errors may result if body composition variables are not measured following the descriptions provided by the researchers who developed the equation.

6. *Was the prediction equation cross-validated on another sample from the population?* In order to determine the validity or predictive accuracy of a body composition equation, it needs to be tested on other samples from the population. This is typically done by dividing the original sample into validation and cross-validation groups. For example, to establish the validity of a new race-specific BIA equation for American Indian women, we tested over 150 subjects (Stolarczyk et al., 1994). The sample was randomly divided into a validation group (N = 100) and cross-validation group (N = 50). First, the predictive equation was developed using the validation sample, and then its validity was tested by using this BIA equation to predict the FFM of the subjects in the cross-validation sample. However, prediction equations, such as this one, need to be cross-validated on additional samples from the population in order to determine their general applicability and worth. In general, prediction equations that have not been cross-validated on the original study sample or on additional samples in other studies should not be used.

7. *What was the size of the correlation ($r_{y,y'}$) between the reference measure (y) and predicted (y') scores (validity coefficient)? What was the size of the SEE when this equation was applied to the cross-validation sample?* In general, an equation with good predictive accuracy should yield a moderately high validity coefficient ($r_{y,y'} > .80$) and an acceptable SEE (Table 1.8). Keep in mind that the SEE represents the degree of deviation of individual scores from the regression line (Figure 1.2).

8. *Was the average predicted score similar to the average reference score for the cross-validation sample?* The prediction equation should yield comparable reference and predicted means. This is tested using a paired t-test. The two means should not differ significantly. A large difference between predicted and reference means indicates that there is a systematic difference (over- or underestimation) between the validation and

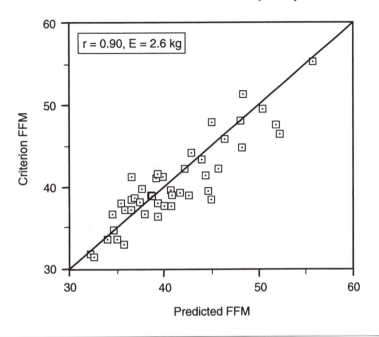

Figure 1.4   Line of identity and total error.

cross-validation samples because of technical error or biological variability (Lohman, 1981).

9. *What was the total error (E) of the equation?* E represents the average deviation of individual scores from the line of identity (Figure 1.4). When an equation closely predicts individual criterion scores, these values will fall closely to the line of identity with a small degree of deviation along this line. When there are small differences between individuals' reference and predicted scores, the total error $[E = \sqrt{\Sigma(y - y')^2/N}]$ will be small. Typically, the E is larger than the SEE because the size of E is affected by both the SEE and the difference between the average predicted and reference scores of the cross-validation sample.

The body composition equations presented in later chapters and in the Quick Reference Guide were selected using the validation and cross-validation principles discussed here. We highly recommend that you apply these criteria when evaluating newly-developed equations or selecting other equations to assess the body composition of your clients.

KEY POINTS

■ Body composition assessment is useful for identifying health risks; determining the health and fitness profiles of your clients; monitoring growth, aging, and disease processes; and evaluating nutrition and exercise interventions.

∎ Although most current body composition prediction equations are based on a two-component body composition model, multicomponent models may yield more accurate prediction equations because these models account for interindividual variation in the water and mineral content of the fat-free body.

∎ Hydrodensitometry and dual-energy x-ray absorptiometry are considered by some experts as the best methods for body composition assessment.

∎ All body composition prediction equations need to be validated and cross-validated to determine their applicability and suitability for use in the field.

∎ Population-specific equations can only be used to estimate the body composition of individuals from a specific group; generalized prediction equations can be used to estimate the body composition of individuals varying in age, gender, race, fatness, or physical activity level.

∎ The relative worth of newly developed body composition methods and prediction equations should be evaluated using specific selection criteria.

Chapter 2

Skinfold Method

In the early 1900s, the thickness of subcutaneous adipose tissue was measured by taking skinfold (SKF) measurements (Brozek & Keys, 1951). Early investigators pointed out that although SKF thicknesses varied at different sites, there were moderate to high relationships among SKF measurements (Brozek & Keys, 1951; Franzen, 1929). Over the years, the SKF method has been widely used to estimate total body fatness in field and clinical settings. Because the SKF test is easy to administer at a relatively low cost, it is suitable for large-scale epidemiological surveys such as the National Health and Nutrition Examination Survey [NHANES III] (Kuczmarski et al., 1994) and clinical nutritional assessment. In addition, SKF measurements are used to estimate regional fat distribution by determining the ratio of subcutaneous fat on the trunk and extremities and to establish anthropometric profiles.

Assumptions and Principles of the Skinfold Method

A SKF indirectly measures the thickness of subcutaneous adipose tissue. Therefore, certain basic relationships are assumed when using the SKF method to estimate total body density to derive relative body fat (%BF).

Assumptions

1. *The SKF is a good measure of subcutaneous fat*. The SKF is a measure of the thickness of two layers of skin and the underlying subcutaneous fat

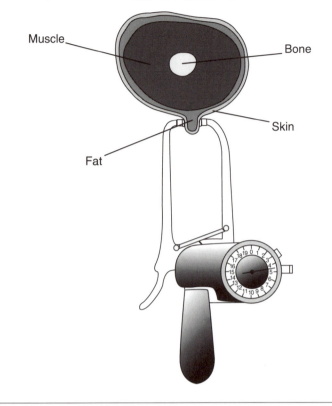

Figure 2.1   Anatomy of a skinfold.

(Figure 2.1). Research has demonstrated that the subcutaneous fat, assessed by SKF measurements at 12 sites, is similar to the value obtained from magnetic resonance imaging (MRI) (Hayes, Sowood, Belyavin, Cohen, & Smith, 1988). However, at some specific sites, SKF measurements yielded significantly smaller amounts of subcutaneous fat compared to that measured directly from MRI (Hayes et al., 1988). This difference may be attributed to the presence of subcutaneous fat below an interface (a layer of irregularity within the fat), thereby limiting the amount of subcutaneous fat that can be lifted in the fold. However, part of this difference also may be due to the distortion of the MRI measurements on the posterior aspect of the body because the subject must be supine in the MRI scanner.

    2. *The distribution of fat subcutaneously and internally is similar for all individuals within each gender.* The validity of this assumption is questionable. Older subjects of the same gender and body density have proportionately less subcutaneous fat than their younger counterparts. Also, the level of body fatness affects the relative amount of fat located internally and subcutaneously. Lean individuals have a higher proportion of internal fat,

and the proportion of fat located internally decreases as overall body fatness increases (Lohman, 1981).

3. *Because there is relationship between subcutaneous fat and total body fat, the sum of several skinfolds can be used to estimate total body fat.* Research has established that SKF thicknesses at multiple sites measure a common body-fat factor (Jackson & Pollock, 1976; Quatrochi et al., 1992). It is assumed that approximately one third of the total fat is located subcutaneously in men and women (Lohman, 1981). However, there is considerable biological variation in subcutaneous, intramuscular, intermuscular, and internal organ fat deposits, as well as essential lipids in bone marrow and the central nervous system. Biological variation in fat distribution is affected by age, gender, and degree of fatness (Lohman, 1981). Therefore, these factors need to be considered in developing prediction equations to estimate relative body fatness.

Principles

1. *There is a relationship between the sum of SKFs (ΣSKF) and body density (Db).* This relationship is linear for homogenous samples (population-specific SKF equations) but nonlinear over a wide range of Db (generalized SKF equations) for both men and women. A linear regression line, depicting the relationship between the ΣSKF and Db, will fit the data well only within a narrow range of body fatness values. Thus, using a population-specific equation to estimate the Db of clients not representative of the sample originally used to develop that equation leads to an inaccurate estimate of your client's Db (Jackson, 1984).

2. *Age is an independent predictor of Db for both men and women.* Using age and the quadratic expression of the sum of skinfolds (ΣSKF^2) accounts for more variance in Db of a heterogeneous population than using the ΣSKF^2 alone (Jackson, 1984).

Skinfold Prediction Models

SKF prediction equations are developed using either linear (population-specific) or quadratic (generalized) regression models. There are over 100 population-specific equations to predict Db from various combinations of SKFs, circumferences, and bony diameters (Jackson & Pollock, 1985). These equations were developed for relatively homogeneous populations and are assumed to be valid only for individuals having similar characteristics, such as age, gender, ethnicity, or level of physical activity. For example, an equation derived specifically for 18- to 21-year-old sedentary men would not be valid for predicting the Db of 35- to 45-year-old sedentary men. Population-specific equations are based on a linear relationship between skinfold fat and Db (linear model);

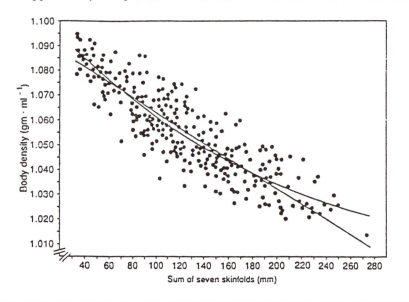

Figure 2.2   Relationship of the sum of skinfolds to body density.
Note. From "Generalized Equations for Predicting Body Density of Men" by A.S. Jackson and M.L. Pollock, 1978, *British Journal of Nutrition*, **40**, p. 502. Copyright 1978 by Cambridge University Press. Reprinted with the permission of Cambridge University Press.

however, research shows that there is a curvilinear relationship (quadratic model) between SKFs and Db across a large range of body fatness (Figure 2.2). Thus, population-specific equations tend to underestimate %BF in fatter subjects and overestimate it in leaner subjects.

Using the quadratic model, generalized equations applicable to individuals varying greatly in age (18 to 60 years) and body fatness (up to 45 %BF) have been developed and validated (Jackson & Pollock, 1978; Jackson, Pollock, & Ward, 1980; Lohman, 1981). These equations also take into account the effect of age on the distribution of subcutaneous and internal fat. An advantage of the generalized equations is that one equation, instead of several, can give accurate estimates of your clients' %BF.

Most equations use two or three SKFs to predict Db. The Db is then converted to %BF using the appropriate population-specific conversion formula (Table 1.6). Boileau, Lohman, and Slaughter (1985) developed SKF equations to predict %BF rather than Db of children (see chapter 6). They determined the reference %BF of these children using a multicomponent body composition model that included measures of body density, total body water, and bone mineral.

Using the Skinfold Method

Commonly-used population-specific and generalized SKF prediction equations are presented in chapters 6 to 10 and are summarized in the Quick

Reference Guide in Appendix A. Calculating the Db and %BF is tedious and time-consuming, especially when you are assessing the body composition of many clients. Therefore, we recommend using the computer software developed for the SKF equations in this book. This software selects the appropriate SKF equation and population-specific conversion formula (Table 1.6) to estimate %BF based on physical demographics (e.g., age, gender, ethnicity, and physical activity level) of your client.

Alternatively, nomograms have been developed for some SKF prediction equations (Figure 2.3). This nomogram was specifically developed for the Jackson sum of three SKF equations. To use this nomogram, the sum of three skinfolds (Σ3SKF) and age is plotted in the appropriate column, and a ruler is used to connect these two points. The corresponding %BF is read at the point where the connecting line intersects the %BF column on the nomogram.

Although nomograms are potential time-savers, you should be aware that this nomogram (Figure 2.3) is based on a two-component body composition model, using the Siri equation to convert Db to %BF. Therefore, in general, you should only use this nomogram to calculate %BF of white males.

Sources of Measurement Error

The validity and reliability of SKF measurements and the SKF method are affected by the *technician's skill, type of SKF caliper, subject factors, and the prediction equation used* to estimate body fatness (Lohman, Pollock, Slaughter, Brandon, & Boileau, 1984). The theoretical accuracy of SKF equations for predicting Db is 0.0075 g/cc or 3.3 %BF due to biological variability in estimating subcutaneous fat from SKF thicknesses and interindividual differences in the relationship between subcutaneous fat and total body fat (Lohman, 1981). Therefore, prediction errors of *≤ 3.5 %BF* or *≤ .0080 g/cc* for SKF equations are acceptable (Table 1.8) because some of this error is attributed to the reference method (Jackson, 1984). To increase the accuracy and precision of your SKF measurements, carefully follow the standardized procedures and guidelines outlined in the SKF technique section of this chapter.

Technician Skill

A major source of error in SKF measurements is variability among technicians. Approximately 3% to 9% of the variability in SKF measurements can be attributed to measurement error due to differences between SKF technicians (Lohman, Pollock, et al., 1984; Morrow, Fridye, & Monaghen, 1986). The amount of between-technician error depends on the site being measured, with larger errors reported for the abdomen (8.8%) and thigh

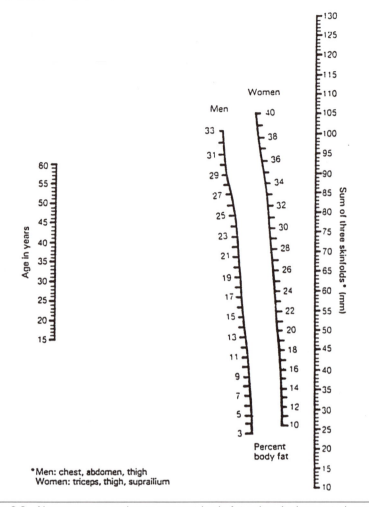

Figure 2.3 Nomogram to estimate percent body fat using Jackson et al. generalized skinfold equations.

Note. From "A Nomogram for the Estimate of Percent Body Fat From Generalized Equations" by W.B. Baun and M.R. Baun, 1981. This figure is reprinted with permission from the *Research Quarterly for Exercise and Sport, 52*, p. 382. *The Research Quarterly for Exercise and Sport* is a publication of the American Alliance for Health, Physical Education, Recreation, and Dance, 1900 Association Drive, Reston, VA 22091.

(7.1%) SKF sites compared to the triceps (~3.0%), subscapular (~3.0% to 5.0%), and suprailiac (~4%) SKF sites (Lohman, Pollock, et al., 1984; Morrow et al., 1986).

Objectivity, or between-technician reliability, is enhanced when SKF technicians *follow standardized testing procedures, practice taking SKFs together, and mark the SKF site* (Pollock & Jackson, 1984). Although some experts believe that SKF sites do not need to be marked (Harrison et al., 1988), we highly recommend doing so, particularly if you are a novice SKF technician. Improperly locating and measuring SKF sites are major causes of low intertester reliability (Lohman, Pollock, et al., 1984). This is most likely due to the lack of standardized site selection and location. For example, Behnke and Wilmore (1974) recommend measuring the abdominal SKF using a horizontal fold adjacent to the umbilicus; whereas, Jackson and Pollock (1978) recommend measuring a vertical fold taken 2 cm lateral to the umbilicus. Inconsistencies like this have led to confusion and lack of agreement among SKF technicians.

As a result, experts in the field of anthropometry have developed standardized testing procedures and detailed descriptions for identification and measurement of SKF sites (Harrison et al., 1988). Some of the most commonly-used sites, described in the *Anthropometric Standardization Reference Manual* (Harrison et al., 1988), are summarized in Table 2.1 and illustrated in Figures 2.4 to 2.12 (see pp. 30-38).

Although the objective is for all SKF technicians to follow standardized procedures and recommendations for site location and SKF measurements, you may not be able to do so in some cases. For example, if you are using the generalized equations of Jackson and Pollock (1978) and Jackson, Pollock, and Ward (1980), the chest, midaxillary, subscapular, abdominal, and suprailiac SKFs will be measured at sites that differ from those described in Table 2.1. The descriptions of the sites used for the Jackson SKF equations are presented in Table 2.2 (see p. 39).

Intratester reliability, or consistency of measurements by the skinfold technician, is another source of error for the SKF method. Measuring SKF thicknesses consistently is difficult in obese clients because the SKF may exceed the maximum aperture of the caliper. Also, in obese and heavily muscled individuals, the subcutaneous fat may not be easily separated from the underlying muscle; therefore, the fold may be more triangular, with sides that are not parallel at the base of the fold (Gray et al., 1990). Thus, proper caliper placement, perpendicular to the fold, is not possible. *Experts recommend practicing your SKF technique on 50 to 100 clients to develop a high level of skill and proficiency* (Jackson & Pollock, 1985; Katch & Katch, 1980). You should take a minimum of two measurements at each site using a rotational order. If SKF values at a given site vary by more than ±10%, you need to take additional measurements. For example, if you initially measure a SKF thickness of 30 mm, values from 27 mm to 33 mm would be acceptable for the second SKF measurement (30 ± 10% or 30 ± 3 mm). The two measurements within ±10% of each other are averaged and used in the prediction equations to estimate Db or %BF.

Type of Caliper

Either high-quality metal calipers or plastic calipers can be used to measure SKF thickness (Figure 2.13, p. 40). The cost of SKF calipers varies, depending

Table 2.1   Standardized Sites for Skinfold Measurements

Site	Direction of fold	Anatomical reference	Measurement
Chest	Diagonal	Axilla and nipple	Fold is taken between axilla and nipple as high as possible on anterior axillary fold with measurement taken 1 cm below fingers.
Subscapular	Diagonal	Inferior angle of scapula	Fold is along natural cleavage line of skin just inferior to inferior angle of scapula, with caliper applied 1 cm below fingers.
Midaxillary	Horizontal	Xiphisternal junction (point where costal cartilage of ribs 5-6 articulate with sternum, slightly above inferior tip of xiphoid process)	Fold is taken on midaxillary line at level of xiphisternal junction.
Suprailiac	Oblique	Iliac crest	Fold is grasped posteriorly to midaxillary line and superiorly to iliac crest along natural cleavage of skin with caliper applied 1 cm below fingers.
Abdominal	Horizontal	Umbilicus	Fold is taken 3 cm lateral and 1 cm inferior to center of the umbilicus.
Triceps	Vertical (midline)	Acromial process of scapula and olecranon process of ulna	Distance between lateral projection of acromial process and inferior margin of olecranon process is measured on lateral aspect of arm with elbow flexed 90° using a tape measure. Midpoint is marked on lateral side of arm. Fold is lifted 1 cm above marked line on posterior aspect of arm. Caliper is applied at marked level.

Site	Direction of fold	Anatomical reference	Measurement
Biceps	Vertical (midline)	Biceps brachii	Fold is lifted over belly of the biceps brachii at the level marked for the triceps and on line with anterior border of the acromial process and the antecubital fossa. Caliper is applied 1 cm below fingers.
Thigh	Vertical (midline)	Inguinal crease and patella	Fold is lifted on anterior aspect of thigh midway between inguinal crease and proximal border of patella. Body weight is shifted to left foot and caliper is applied 1 cm below fingers.
Calf	Vertical (medial aspect)	Maximal calf circumference	Fold is lifted at level of maximal calf circumference on medial aspect of calf with knee and hip flexed to 90°.

Note. Adapted from Harrison et al. (1988, pp. 55-70).

on the materials used in construction (metal or plastic) and the caliper's accuracy and precision throughout the range of measurement. High-quality instruments, such as Harpenden, Lange, Holtain, and Lafayette calipers, exert constant pressure (~10 g/mm^2) throughout the range of measurement (0 mm to 60 mm). Calipers should not vary in tension more than 2.0 g/mm^2 over the range or exceed 15 g/mm^2 (Edwards, Hammond, Healy, Tanner, & Whitehouse, 1955). Excessive tension and force cause client discomfort (a pinching sensation) and significantly reduce the SKF measurement (Gruber, Pollock, Graves, Colvin, & Braith, 1990). High-quality calipers also have excellent scale precision (0.2 mm and 1.0 mm for Harpenden and Lange calipers, respectively). *The accuracy of your caliper should be checked periodically using a high precision vernier caliper or SKF calibration blocks* (see Appendix B for manufacturer's address). To calibrate the SKF caliper with a vernier caliper, set the opening of the vernier caliper to a given width (e.g., 20 mm) and place the jaws of the SKF caliper on it. The value read from the SKF caliper (20 mm) should match the preset width of the vernier caliper. If it does not, follow the manufacturer's calibration instructions or send the SKF caliper to the manufacturer for recalibration.

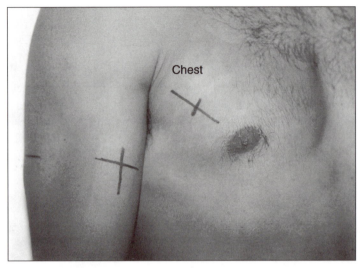

a

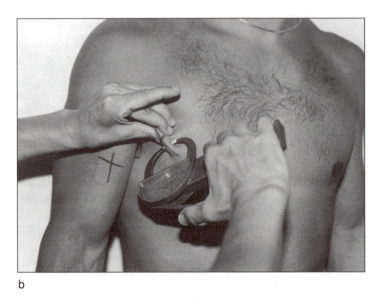

b

Figure 2.4   (a) Site and (b) measurement of the chest skinfold.

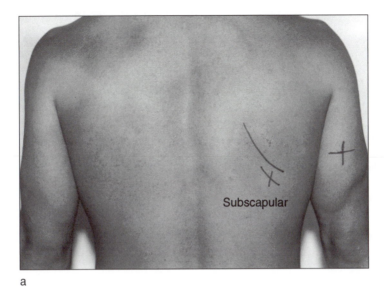

Subscapular

a

b

Figure 2.5 (a) Site and (b) measurement of the subscapular skinfold.

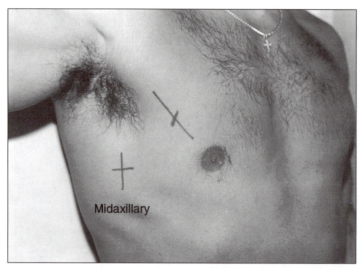

a

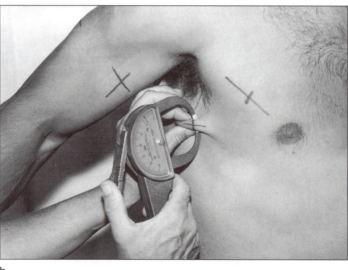

b

Figure 2.6   (a) Site and (b) measurement of the midaxillary skinfold.

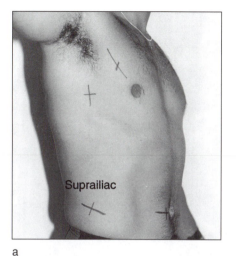

a

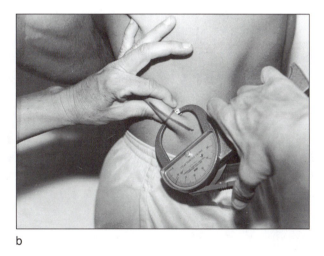

b

Figure 2.7   (a) Site and (b) measurement of the suprailiac skinfold.

Although the Harpenden and Lange SKF calipers have similar pressure characteristics, a number of researchers reported that SKFs measured with Harpenden calipers produce significantly smaller values compared to Lange calipers (Gruber et al., 1990; Lohman, Pollock, et al., 1984). This difference translates into a systematic underestimation (~1.5 %BF) of average %BF for women and men when using the Harpenden calipers (Gruber et al., 1990). Even though the pressure is similar for the Lange (9.3 g/mm^2) and Harpenden

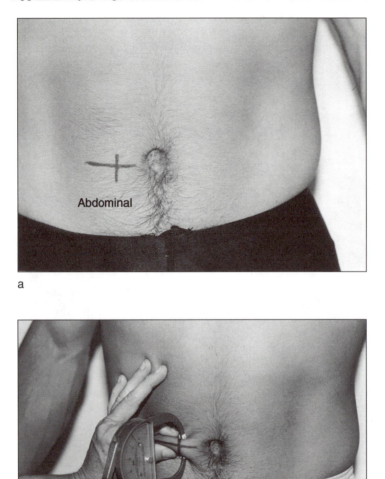

a

b

Figure 2.8 (a) Site and (b) measurement of the abdominal skinfold.

(9.36 g/mm^2) calipers, researchers noted that the Harpenden caliper requires three times more force to open its jaws. Therefore, it is more likely

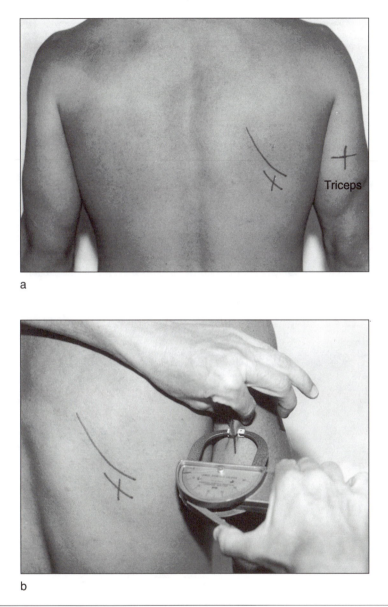

Figure 2.9   (a) Site and (b) measurement of the triceps skinfold.

that the adipose tissue will be compressed to a greater extent, resulting in smaller SKF measurements with this type of caliper.

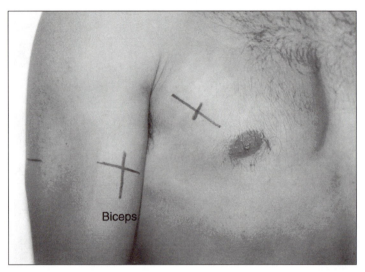

a

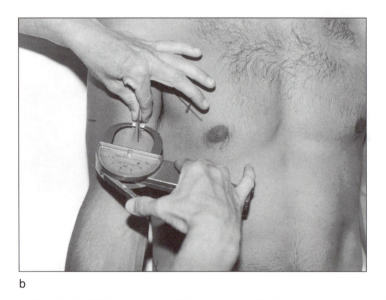

b

Figure 2.10   (a) Site and (b) measurement of the biceps skinfold.

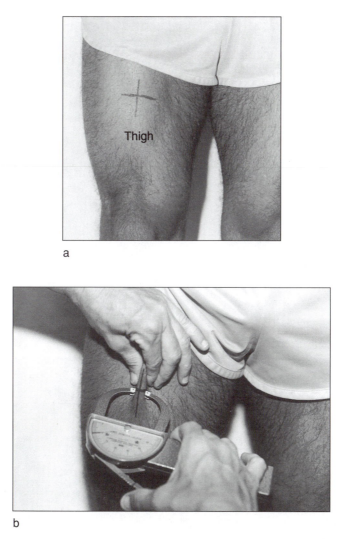

a

b

Figure 2.11   (a) Site and (b) measurement of the thigh skinfold.

Compared to high-quality calipers, plastic SKF calipers have

a. less scale precision (~2 mm),
b. nonconstant tension throughout the range of measurement (Hawkins, 1983),
c. smaller measurement scale (~40 mm), and
d. less consistency when used by inexperienced SKF technicians (Lohman, Pollock, et al., 1984).

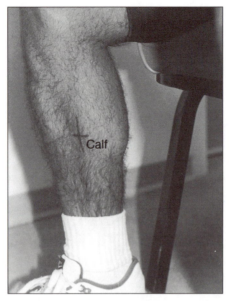

a

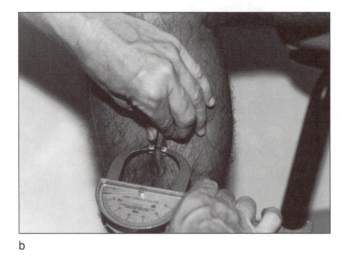

b

Figure 2.12 (a) Site and (b) measurement of the calf skinfold.

Table 2.2   Skinfold Sites for Jackson's Generalized Skinfold Equations

Site	Direction of fold	Anatomical reference	Measurement
Chest	Diagonal	Axilla and nipple	Fold is taken 1/2 the distance between the anterior axillary line and nipple for men and 1/3 of this distance for women.
Subscapular	Oblique	Vertebral border and inferior angle of scapula	Fold is taken on diagonal line coming from the vertebral border, 1-2 cm below the inferior angle.
Midaxillary	Vertical	Xiphoid process of sternum	Fold is taken at level of xiphoid process along the midaxillary line.
Suprailiac	Diagonal	Iliac crest	Fold is taken diagonally above the iliac crest along the anterior axillary line.
Abdominal	Vertical	Umbilicus	Fold is taken vertically 2 cm lateral to the umbilicus.

Note. Adapted from Jackson and Pollock (1978) and Jackson et al. (1980).

Despite these differences, a number of researchers (Hawkins, 1983; Leger, Lambert, & Martin, 1982; Lohman, Pollock, et al., 1984) reported no significant differences between SKFs measured with high-quality calipers (Harpenden, Holtain, and Lange) and plastic calipers (McGaw caliper, Ross adipometer, and Fat-O-Meter). Others have found that SKFs measured with Harpenden, McGaw, Slim-Guide, and Skyndex calipers are significantly smaller than those measured with Lange calipers (Burgert & Anderson, 1979; Gruber et al., 1990; Hawkins, 1983; Lohman, Pollock, et al., 1984; Zando & Robertson, 1987). Lohman, Pollock, et al. (1984) noted that differences among instruments (Harpenden, Lange, Holtain, and Ross adipometer calipers) varied depending on the SKF technician. Differences among technicians were less for the Harpenden and Holtain calipers compared to the Lange caliper and Ross adipometer. Given that the caliper's type may be a potential source of measurement error, *we recommend that you use the same caliper when monitoring changes in your client's SKF thicknesses.*

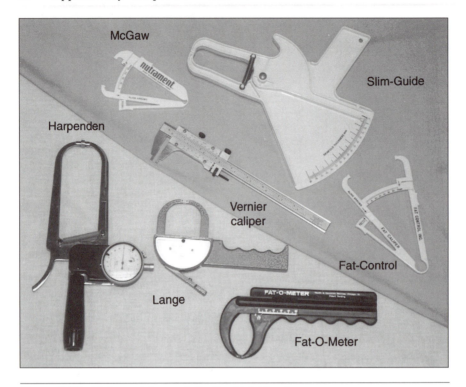

Figure 2.13 High-precision and plastic skinfold calipers.

Subject Factors

Variability in SKF measurements among individuals may be attributed not only to differences in the amount of subcutaneous fat at the site, but to differences in *skin thickness, compressibility of the adipose tissue, handedness, and hydration levels* of your clients. Interindividual variability in skin thickness (0.5 mm to 2 mm) is small and does not contribute substantially to the total measurement error for SKF thicknesses (Keys & Brozek, 1953). However, Martin, Drinkwater, and Clarys (1992) reported that variation in SKF compressibility may be an important limitation of the SKF method.

An accumulation of extracellular water (edema) in the subcutaneous tissue caused by factors such as peripheral vasodilation or certain diseases may increase skinfold thicknesses (Keys & Brozek, 1953). This suggests that *SKFs should not be measured immediately after exercise*, especially in hot environments. Also, most of the weight gain experienced by some women during their menstrual cycles is caused by water retention (Bunt, Lohman, & Boileau, 1989). This could increase SKF thicknesses, particularly on the trunk and abdomen. However, there are no empirical data to support or refute this hypothesis. Also, subcutaneous edema induced intravenously has an effect on skinfold measurements and the pliability of the skin (Grant, Custer, & Thurlaw, 1981).

Finally, for some individuals, there may be a difference in the size of SKFs taken on the right and left sides of the body due to the handedness of the individual (Damon, 1965; Martorell, Mendoza, Mueller, & Pawson, 1988). However, the average difference between triceps SKFs on the right and left arms (0.5 mm) was quite small (Martorell et al., 1988). Still there is a lack of standardization as to which side of the body anthropometric measurements should be taken. In the United States, researchers generally take these measurements on the right side of the body, as recommended in the *Anthropometric Standardization Reference Manual* (Harrison et al., 1988). On the other hand, the general practice in Europe and developing countries is to measure SKFs on the left side of the body, as recommended by the International Biological Programs (Martorell et al., 1988). By following the standardized procedures and guidelines outlined in the SKF technique section of this chapter, measurement error due to subject factors can be controlled.

Skinfold Prediction Equations

As mentioned earlier in this chapter, SKF prediction equations should be selected based on the age, gender, ethnicity, and physical activity level of your client. Lohman, Pollock, et al. (1984) compared %BF estimates obtained from five different SKF prediction equations applied to a sample of female, collegiate basketball players. Four of these equations were developed and cross-validated on female, nonathletic populations; whereas, the fifth equation was developed specifically for female athletes. The average %BF estimates ranged from 16.5% (the athlete's equation) to 24.2%, illustrating the necessity of selecting the appropriate equation in order to obtain the best estimate of your client's body fatness. Given that this is a major source of measurement error, the SKF equations recommended in later chapters have been carefully selected based on research substantiating their applicability for estimating levels of body fat for specific population subgroups.

Skinfold Technique

It takes a great deal of time and practice to develop your skill as a SKF technician. Following standardized procedures will increase the accuracy and reliability of your measurements (Harrison et al., 1988):

1. Take all SKF measurements on the right side of the body.
2. Carefully identify, measure, and mark the SKF site, especially if you are a novice SKF technician (see Figures 2.4 to 2.12).

3. Grasp the SKF firmly between the thumb and index finger of your left hand. The fold is lifted 1 cm above the site to be measured.
4. Lift the fold by placing the thumb and index finger 8 cm (~3 inches) apart on a line that is perpendicular to the long axis of the skinfold. The long axis is parallel to the natural cleavage lines of the skin. However, for individuals with extremely large skinfolds, the thumb and finger will need to be separated more than 8 cm in order to lift the fold.
5. Keep the fold elevated while the measurement is taken.
6. Place the jaws of the caliper perpendicular to the fold, approximately 1 cm below the thumb and index finger, and release the jaw pressure slowly.
7. Take the SKF measurement 4 seconds after the pressure is released.
8. Open the jaws of the caliper to remove it from the site. Close the jaws slowly to prevent damage or loss of calibration.

You will also be able to increase your skill as a skinfold technician by following these recommendations made by experts in the field (Jackson & Pollock, 1985; Lohman, Pollock, et al., 1984; Pollock & Jackson, 1984):

- Be meticulous when locating the anatomical landmarks used to identify the SKF site, when measuring the distance, and when marking the site with a surgical marking pen.
- Read the dial of the caliper to the nearest 0.1 mm (Harpenden or Holtain), 0.5 mm (Lange), or 1 mm (plastic calipers).
- Take a minimum of two measurements at each site. If values vary from each other by more than ±10%, take additional measurements.
- Take skinfold measurements in a rotational order (circuits) rather than consecutive readings at each site.
- Take the SKF measurements when the client's skin is dry and lotion-free.
- Do not measure SKFs immediately after exercise because the shift in body fluid to the skin tends to increase the size of the SKF.
- Practice taking SKFs on 50 to 100 clients.
- Avoid using plastic calipers if you are an inexperienced SKF technician.
- Train with skilled SKF technicians, and compare your results.
- Use a SKF training videotape that demonstrates proper SKF techniques (Lohman, 1987).
- Seek additional training at workshops held at state, regional, and national conferences.

As you can surmise, it takes much practice and patience to become a skilled SKF technician. In certain cases, even highly skilled technicians will be unable to accurately measure the SKF thicknesses of extremely obese or heavily muscled individuals. For these clients, alternative methods, such as BIA, can be used to assess body fatness.

KEY POINTS

▮ The ΣSKF is a good measure of subcutaneous adipose tissue and can be used to estimate total body fatness.

▮ The ΣSKF is inversely related to total Db and directly related to %BF.

▮ Population-specific SKF equations are based on a linear model and are applicable only to individuals from a specific population subgroup. Generalized SKF equations are based on a quadratic model and are applicable to individuals who vary greatly in age and level of body fatness.

▮ Select the appropriate SKF equation for each client. Key equations are highlighted in chapters 6 through 10 and summarized in the Quick Reference Guide.

▮ A major source of measurement error for the SKF method is the technician's skill in locating and measuring the SKF.

▮ Following standardized procedures will increase the accuracy and precision of SKF measurements. Use of SKF training videotapes and workshops is an essential part of the standardization process.

▮ Practice and training with experienced technicians are keys to becoming a skilled SKF technician.

Chapter 3

Bioelectrical Impedance Method

Bioelectrical impedance analysis (BIA) is a rapid, noninvasive, and relatively inexpensive method for evaluating body composition in field and clinical settings. Thomasett's (1962) pioneering work in the early 1960s established basic BIA principles. With this method, low-level electrical current is passed through the client's body, and the impedance (Z), or opposition to the flow of current, is measured with a BIA analyzer. The individual's total body water (TBW) can be estimated from the impedance measurement because the electrolytes in the body's water are excellent conductors of electrical current. When the volume of TBW is large, the current flows more easily through the body with less resistance (R). The resistance to current flow will be greater in individuals with large amounts of body fat, given that adipose tissue is a poor conductor of electrical current due to its relatively small water content. Because the water content of the fat-free body is relatively large (73% water), fat-free mass (FFM) can be predicted from TBW estimates. Individuals with a large FFM and TBW have less resistance to current flowing through their bodies, compared to those having a smaller fat-free mass.

Hoffer, Meador, and Simpson (1969) reported a strong relationship between total body impedance measures and TBW, suggesting that the BIA method may be a valuable tool for analyzing body composition and assessing TBW in the clinical setting. In addition to the research substantiating that TBW can be estimated from impedance measures with a fair degree of accuracy (Kushner & Schoeller, 1992; Lukaski & Bolonchuk, 1988; Van Loan et al., 1990; Van Loan & Mayclin, 1987), other researchers demonstrated that FFM or relative body fat (%BF) could also be accurately predicted in children and adults using the BIA method (Deurenberg, van der Kooy, Leenan, Westrate, & Seidell, 1991; Houtkooper, Lohman, Going, & Hall, 1989; Lukaski, Johnson, Bolonchuk, & Lykken, 1985; Segal, Gutin, Presta, Wang, & Van Itallie, 1985; Segal, Van Loan, Fitzgerald, Hodgdon, & Van Itallie, 1988; Van Loan & Mayclin, 1987).

Although the relative predictive accuracy of the BIA method is similar to the SKF method, BIA may be preferable in some settings because

a. it does not require a high degree of technician skill,
b. it is generally more comfortable and does not intrude as much upon the client's privacy, and
c. it can be used to estimate body composition of obese individuals (Gray, Bray, Gemayel, & Kaplan, 1989; Segal et al., 1988).

BIA has the potential to assess regional body composition, particularly the soft tissue composition of the trunk (Going, Lohman, Williams, Hewitt, & Haber, 1989). Additionally, with multifrequency bioelectrical impedance analysis, it may soon be possible to estimate extracellular water and intracellular water compartments, along with TBW (Espejo et al., 1989; Segal et al., 1991; Van Loan, Withers, Matthie, & Mayclin, 1993). Potentially, this could enhance the clinical application of BIA to assess changes and shifts between the intracellular water and extracellular water compartments associated with certain diseases. For an excellent overview of BIA and its applications, we recommend reading Baumgartner, Chumlea, and Roche (1990); Kushner (1992); Lukaski (1987); and Van Loan (1990).

Assumptions and Principles of the BIA Method

The volume of the body's FFM or TBW is indirectly estimated from bioelectrical impedance measures. Therefore, certain basic assumptions about the geometric shape of the body and the relationship of impedance to the length and volume of the conductor are made.

Assumptions

1. *The human body is shaped like a perfect cylinder with a uniform length and cross-sectional area.* This assumption is not entirely true. As illustrated in Figure 3.1, the human body more closely depicts five cylinders (two arms, two legs, and trunk, excluding the head) connected in a series, instead of one large, perfect cylinder (Kushner, 1992). Because the body segments are

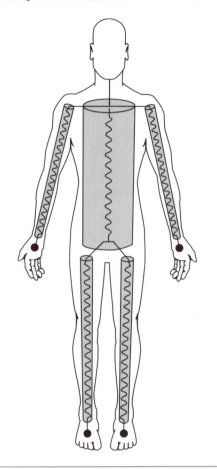

Figure 3.1   Five-cylinder model connected in electrical series.
Note. From "Bioelectrical Impedance Analysis: A Review of Principles and Applications" by R.F. Kushner, 1992, *Journal of the American College of Nutrition,* **11**, p. 201. Copyright 1992 by American College of Nutrition. Reprinted with permission.

not uniform in length or cross-sectional area, resistance to the flow of current through these body segments will differ.

2. *Assuming the body is a perfect cylinder, at a fixed signal frequency (e.g., 50 kHz), the impedance (Z) to current flow through the body is directly related to the length (L) of the conductor (height) and inversely related to its cross-sectional area (A): Z = p(L/A),* where p is the specific resistivity of the body's tissues and is assumed to be constant. To express this relationship in terms of Z and the body's volume, instead of its cross-sectional area, the equation is multiplied by L/L: $Z = p(L/A)(L/L)$. A × L is equal to volume (V), so rearranging this equation yields $V = pL^2/Z$. Thus, the volume of the FFM or TBW of the body is directly related to L^2, or height squared (HT^2), and indirectly related to Z.

However, the application of this equation may not be perfect because of the complex geometric shape of the body (Van Loan, 1990). Also, specific resistivity (*p*) is not constant and has been shown to vary among body segments because of differences in tissue composition, hydration levels, and electrolyte concentration (Kushner, 1992). Chumlea, Baumgartner, and Roche (1988) reported that the specific resistivity of the trunk is two to three times greater than that of the extremities. Also, the specific resistivity of the arms and legs is greater in adults compared to children and in obese compared to normal-weight individuals (Chumlea et al., 1988; Fuller & Elia, 1989).

Principles

1. *Biological tissues act as conductors or insulators, and the flow of current through the body will follow the path of least resistance.* Because the FFM contains large amounts of water (~73%) and electrolytes, it is a better conductor of electrical current than fat. To measure total body impedance, a low-level excitation current (500 µA to 800 µA) at 50kHz is used. At low frequencies (~1 kHz), the current passes through the extracellular fluids only; at higher frequencies (500 kHz to 800 kHz), it penetrates cell membranes and passes through the intracellular fluid, as well as the extracellular fluid (Lukaski, 1987). Given that fat is anhydrous and a poor conductor of electrical current, the total body impedance, measured at the constant frequency of 50 kHz, primarily reflects the volumes of the water and muscle compartments comprising the FFM and the extracellular water volume (Kushner, 1992).

2. *Impedance is a function of resistance and reactance, where* $Z = \sqrt{(R^2 + X_c^2)}$. Resistance (R) is a measure of pure opposition to current flow through the body; reactance (X_c) is the opposition to current flow caused by capacitance produced by the cell membrane (Kushner, 1992). The size of R is much larger than X_c (at a 50 kHz frequency) when measuring whole body impedance; therefore, R is a better predictor of FFM and TBW than Z (Lohman, 1989b). For these reasons, the resistance index (HT^2/R), instead of HT^2/Z, is often used in many BIA models to predict FFM or TBW (Lohman, 1989b). However, Lukaski and Bolonchuk (1988) noted that HT^2/X_c was a better predictor of extracellular water than HT^2/R. Segal, Kral, Wang, Pierson, & Van Itallie (1987) reported that X_c was strongly related to the ratio of extracellular to intracellular water and was able to discriminate between subjects with normal and abnormal hydration levels.

BIA Prediction Models

BIA prediction equations are based on either population-specific or generalized models. These equations estimate FFM and TBW because of theoretical and empirical relationships established among FFM, TBW, and bio-impedance measures. Many population-specific BIA equations have been developed for homogenous subgroups to account for differences due to age, ethnicity, gender, physical activity level, and level of body fatness. Therefore, these equations are valid for and can only be applied to individuals whose physical characteristics are similar to those in the specific population subgroup. For example, an equation developed for younger men (18 to 30 years) will systematically overestimate the FFM of older men (60 to 83 years) because the intercepts (I) of the regression lines are different for younger (I = 10.9) and older (I = 7.0) men (Deurenberg, van der Kooy, Evers, & Hulshof, 1990). This demonstrates that the relationship between the resistance index (HT^2/R) and FFM is highly dependent on age. Similarly, other researchers have reported that the predictive accuracy of the BIA method may be improved using age-specific (Lohman, 1992), race-specific (Rising, Swinburn, Larson, & Ravussin, 1991; Stolarczyk et al., 1994), fatness-specific (Gray et al., 1989; Segal et al., 1988), and physical-activity-level-specific (Houtkooper, Going, Westfall, & Lohman, 1989) equations.

As an alternative to population-specific equations, generalized BIA equations developed for heterogeneous populations varying in age, gender, and body fatness, can be used. This approach accounts for the biological variability among population subgroups by including factors such as age and gender as predictor variables in BIA equations estimating FFM or TBW (Deurenberg, van der Kooy, Evers, & Hulshof, 1990; Gray et al., 1989; Kushner & Schoeller, 1986; Lukaski & Bolonchuk, 1988; Van Loan & Mayclin, 1987).

Regardless of the approach (population-specific or generalized), the predictive accuracy of BIA equations typically is improved by including body weight, along with HT^2 and R, in the BIA regression model. The human body is not a perfect cylinder with a uniform cross-sectional area, and the specific resistivity of tissues is not constant. Thus, including body weight in the equation may be one way of accounting for the complex geometric shape of the body, as well as individual differences in trunk size (Kushner, 1992). Generally, the resistance index, HT^2/R, is a relatively stronger predictor of FFM than body weight (Lohman, 1992). Most BIA equations use either HT^2/R or HT^2 and R separately as predictors of FFM.

Although X$_c$ is not typically included as a predictor in most BIA equations, it is moderately related to relative body fatness. X$_c$ may reflect changes in fluid distribution and hydration of adipose tissue and FFM associated with increased fatness (Baumgartner, Chumlea, & Roche, 1988). In fact, we recently published a BIA equation for a sample of American Indian women with an average body fatness of 37 %BF. In this equation, X$_c$ accounted for a significant proportion of the variance in FFM, in addition to HT^2, R, body weight, and age (Stolarczyk et al., 1994).

To date there are only a few BIA equations using multicomponent models to derive reference measures of FFM (Guo, Roche, & Houtkooper, 1989; Houtkooper, Going, Lohman, Roche, & Van Loan, 1992; Lohman, 1992;

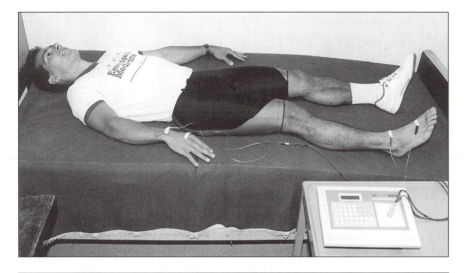

Figure 3.2 BIA electrode placement and client positioning.

Stolarczyk et al., 1994; Van Loan et al., 1990). This research suggests that the predictive accuracy of the BIA method may be improved when a multi-component model is used, particularly for population subgroups whose fat-free body composition differs from the assumed values of the two-component model (e.g., American Indians, elderly, and children).

Using the BIA Method

The tetrapolar method uses four electrodes applied to the hand, wrist, foot, and ankle (Figure 3.2). An excitation current of (500 µA to 800 µA) at 50 kHz is applied at the source (distal) electrodes on the hand and foot, and the voltage drop due to impedance is detected by the sensor (proximal) electrodes on the wrist and ankle.

Commonly used, population-specific and generalized BIA equations are presented in chapters 6 to 10 and summarized in the Quick Reference Guide. To use these equations, R and X_c are obtained directly from your BIA analyzer. The complementary computer software allows you to select an appropriate BIA equation to estimate your client's FFM based on physical characteristics (i.e., age, gender, race, physical activity level, and level of body fatness). Using this software will save time and prevent errors in calculating FFM from these equations. The %BF of your client is estimated by determining the fat mass (FM = BW − FFM) and dividing FM by the client's body weight [%BF = (FM/BW) × 100].

At this time, *we do not recommend using the FFM and %BF estimates obtained directly from your BIA analyzer* (BMR, Holtain, RJL, or Valhalla) unless you

a. know which equations are programmed in the analyzer's computer software,
b. obtain information from the manufacturer regarding the validity and accuracy of these equations, and
c. determine if these equations are generalizable and applicable to your clients.

Sources of Measurement Error

The accuracy and precision of the BIA method are affected by *instrumentation, subject factors, technician skill, environmental factors, and the prediction equation used to estimate FFM* (Kushner, 1992; Lohman, 1989b; Van Loan, 1990). The theoretical error is estimated to be ~1.8 kg, if the reference method (e.g., hydrodensitometry) is error-free (Lohman, 1992). Unfortunately, this is not the case; so part (20% to 50%) of the total prediction error associated with the BIA method and the equations can be attributed to error in the reference method. Therefore, a SEE of ≤ *3.5 kg* for men and ≤ *2.8 kg* for women is acceptable (Table 1.8).

Instrumentation

Although there are a number of fixed-frequency BIA analyzers, two commonly-used impedance analyzers are the RJL System (Detroit, MI) and Valhalla Scientific (San Diego, CA). These analyzers differ in a few ways:

a. The RJL analyzer delivers an alternating current of 800 µA at a fixed 50 kHz frequency; whereas, the Valhalla analyzer uses a 500 µA alternating current at the same, fixed frequency (50 kHz).
b. The BIA equations used in these two types of analyzers not only differ, but also vary from instrument to instrument, depending on the software version programmed into the analyzer; it is important to find out from the manufacturer which equations are in your analyzer.
c. The Valhalla analyzer is calibrated internally with a 499 ohm (Ω) resistor by pressing the calibration key of the analyzer; the RJL analyzer is calibrated externally by attaching a 499 ohm (Ω) resistor to the lead wires.

At present, there are two multifrequency bioimpedance analyzers. The tri-frequency analyzer (Daninger Medical Technology, Columbus, OH) measures R and X_c at three fixed frequencies (5, 50, and 100 kHz). The Xitron

4000 (Xitron Technolgies, San Diego, CA) generates radio frequencies ranging from 1 kHz to 1 MHz. This multifrequency analyzer costs almost twice as much as fixed frequency analyzers and is being marketed only for research purposes at this time.

Research demonstrates that the whole body resistance measured by different brands of single frequency analyzers differs by as much as 36 Ω (Graves, Pollock, Colvin, Van Loan, & Lohman, 1989). For example, the average %BF estimated for men from one BIA equation differed by 6.3 %BF using the Valhalla and Bioelectrical Sciences (BES, La Jolla, CA) analyzers to measure R, and the correlation between resistance values measured with the Valhalla and BES analyzers was only r = 0.59. In comparison, there was a high correlation (r = 0.99) between resistance values obtained with the Valhalla and RJL analyzers. In general, the Valhalla analyzer produced significantly higher resistances than the RJL analyzer for men (~16 Ω) and women (~19 Ω), corresponding to a systematic underestimate of FFM in men (~1.3 kg) and women (~1.0 kg) (Graves et al., 1989). Deurenberg, van der Kooy, and Leenan (1989) reported that instrumentation is a significant source of measurement error. The Z values from three RJL Model 101 analyzers differed by 7 to 16 Ω for their subjects, which corresponded to a difference in FFM of 2.1 kg for some individuals.

Instrumentation is a substantial source of error and one limitation of the BIA method. To control for this error, *the same instrument should be used when monitoring changes in your client's body composition.* The BIA analyzer should be calibrated prior to measuring your client's body composition.

Subject Factors

A major source of error with the BIA method is intra-individual variability in whole body resistance due to factors that alter the client's state of hydration. Between 3.1% and 3.9% of the variance in resistance may be attributed to day-to-day fluctuations in body water (Jackson, Pollock, Graves, & Mahar, 1988). *Factors such as eating, drinking, dehydrating, and exercising alter the individual's hydration state, thereby affecting total body resistance and the estimate of FFM* (Table 3.1). Taking resistance measures 2 to 4 hours after a meal decreases R as much as 13 to 17 Ω and is likely to overpredict the FFM of your client by almost 1.5 kg (Deurenberg, Weststrate, Paymans, & van der Kooy, 1988). However, Rising et al. (1991) reported only small changes in resistances measured one hour before and one hour after eating breakfast or consuming 700 ml of water or diet soda. In contrast, Gomez, Mole, and Collins (1993) noted that resistance increases (~10 Ω) significantly and remains elevated 4 to 90 min after drinking 1 l of water. Lukaski (1986) reported that dehydration increases resistance (~40 Ω), resulting in a 5.0 kg underestimate of FFM.

The effect of aerobic exercise on resistance measurements is partially dependent on exercise intensity and duration. Jogging and cycling at moderate

Table 3.1   Summary of Factors Affecting Bioelectrical Impedance Measures

Factor	Effect on resistance (Ω)	Effect on FFM (kg)	Reference
Type of analyzer *Valhalla vs. RJL*	↑ 16-18[a]	↓ 1.0-1.3	Graves et al. (1989)
Eating or drinking within 4 hr	↑ 13-17	↓ 1.5	Deurenberg et al. (1988)
Dehydration	↑ 40	↓ 5.0	Lukaski (1986)
Aerobic exercise			
Low intensity	NC	NC	Deurenberg et al. (1988)
Moderate-high intensity	↓ 50-70	↑ 12.0	Khaled et al. (1988) Lukaski (1986)
Menstrual cycle			
Follicular vs. premenstrual	↓ 5-8[b]	NC	Gleichauf & Rose (1989)
Menses vs. follicular	↑ 7[c]	NC	
Electrode placement	↑ 10	NC	Elsen et al. (1987)
	↑ 70	11	Lukaski (1986)
Electrode configuration			
Ipsilateral vs. contralateral	NC	NC	Lukaski et al. (1985)
Right side vs. left side	NC	NC	Graves et al. (1989)
Room temperature *14 °C vs. 35 °C*	↑ 35[d]	↓ 2.2	Caton et al. (1988)

NC = no change

[a]Valhalla > RJL

[b]Follicular > premenstrual

[c]Menses > follicular

[d]14 °C > 35 °C

intensities (~70% $\dot{V}O_2$max) for 90 to 120 minutes produced substantial decreases (50 Ω to 70 Ω) in R, resulting in a large overestimate of FFM (~12 kg) (Khaled et al., 1988; Lukaski, 1986). In contrast, cycling at relatively lower intensities (100 and 175 W) for 90 minutes had a much smaller effect (1 Ω to 9 Ω) (Durenberg et al., 1988). The decrease in R after strenuous exercise most likely reflects the relatively greater loss of body water in the sweat and expired air, compared to the loss of electrolytes. This leads to a higher electrolyte concentration in the body's fluids, thereby lowering R values (Deurenberg et al., 1988). Increases in core body temperature and skin temperature may contribute to the sharp decrease in R after exercising because it has been shown that increased skin temperature (33.4 °C compared to 24 °C) decreases R (Caton, Mole, Adams, & Heustis, 1988).

Although the menstrual cycle alters intracellular water, TBW, the ratio of extracellular to intracellular water and body weight (Mitchell, Rose, Familoni, Winters, & Ling, 1993), there are only small changes in bioimpedance measures (Z and R) between the follicular and premenstrual stages (~5 to 8 Ω) and between menses and the follicular stage (~7 Ω) (Deurenberg et al., 1988; Gleichauf & Rose, 1989). However, the average body weight of these women was stable (<0.2 kg) during the menstrual cycle. In women experiencing relatively large body weight gains (2 to 4 kg) during the menstrual cycle, a large part of this weight gain is due to an increase (1.5 kg on average) in TBW (Bunt et al., 1989). Until there are more conclusive data dealing with this issue, *we recommend taking BIA measurements at a time during the menstrual cycle when the client perceives that she is not experiencing a large weight gain.* This practice should minimize error and yield a more accurate estimate of FFM for your clients.

Technician Skill

Technician skill is not a major source of measurement error. There is virtually no difference in R measurements taken by different technicians, provided that standardized procedures for electrode placement and client positioning are closely followed (Jackson et al., 1988). *The proximal sensor electrodes, in particular, need to be correctly positioned at the wrist and ankle.* A 1 cm displacement of the sensor electrodes may result in a 2% error in R (Elsen, Siu, Pineda, & Solomons, 1987). Lukaski (1986) reported a 16% increase in R (~79 Ω) due to improper electrode placement.

As a standard practice, *bioimpedance measures are taken on the right side of the body.* The differences between R measurements using ipsilateral (right arm-right leg or left arm-left leg) and contralateral (right arm-left leg or left arm-right leg) electrode placements are generally small (Graves et al., 1989; Lukaski et al., 1985). *The BIA technician must be certain that the client is lying in a supine position with arms and legs comfortably apart, at about a 45° angle to each other.*

Environmental Factors

Bioimpedance measurements should be made with the client lying supine on a nonconductive surface (e.g., stretcher bed or mat) in a room with normal ambient temperature (35 °C). Cool, ambient temperatures (~14 °C) cause a drop in skin temperature (24 °C, compared to 33 °C under normal conditions), resulting in a significant increase in total body R (+35 Ω, on average) and a decrease in estimated FFM (~2.2 kg) (Caton et al., 1988).

Table 3.2   BIA Client Guidelines

- No eating or drinking within 4 hours of the test.
- No exercise within 12 hours of the test.
- Urinate within 30 minutes of the test.
- No alcohol consumption within 48 hours of the test.
- No diuretic medications within 7 days of the test.
- No testing of female clients who perceive they are retaining water during that stage of their menstrual cycle.

BIA Prediction Equations

BIA prediction equations should be selected based on the age, gender, ethnicity, physical activity level, and level of body fatness of your client. Use of inappropriate equations can lead to systematic prediction errors in estimating FFM. This is a major potential source of error for the BIA method. The BIA equations recommended in later chapters were carefully selected based on research substantiating their applicability and generalizability to specific population subgroups.

BIA Technique

As you can surmise, the accuracy of the bioelectrical impedance (BIA) method is highly dependent on controlling factors that may increase the measurement error of this method. Therefore, it is important to ascertain whether or not your client meets all BIA guidelines (Table 3.2), and follows standardized testing procedures.

1. Bioimpedance measures are taken on the right side of the body with the client lying supine on a nonconductive surface in a room with normal ambient temperature (~35 °C).
2. Clean the skin at the electrode sites with an alcohol pad.
3. Place the sensor (proximal) electrodes (Figure 3.3) on (a) the dorsal surface of the wrist so that the upper border of the electrode bisects the head of the ulna, and (b) the dorsal surface of the ankle so that the upper border of the electrode bisects the medial and lateral malleoli. A measuring tape and surgical marking pen can be used to mark these points for electrode placement.
4. Place the source (distal) electrodes at the base of the second or third metacarpal-phalangeal joints of the hand and foot (Figure 3.3). Make certain there is at least 5 cm between the proximal and distal electrodes.

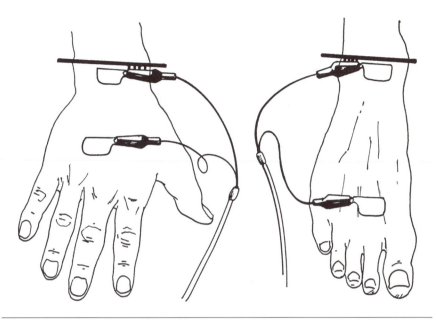

Figure 3.3   Proximal and distal electrode placement.

5. Attach the lead wires to the appropriate electrodes. Red leads are attached to the wrist and ankle, and black leads are attached to the hand and foot.

6. Make certain that the client's legs and arms are abducted approximately 45° to each other. There should be no contact between the thighs and between the arms and the trunk.

KEY POINTS

▌ BIA is a rapid, noninvasive, and nonintrusive method for measuring body composition.

▌ Impedance to current flow through the body is directly related to the square of the individual's height and indirectly related to cross-sectional area.

▌ FFM, with its water and electrolytes, is a good conductor of electrical current; fat is a poor conductor. Therefore, BIA equations can be used to estimate FFM and TBW.

▌ Population-specific BIA equations are applicable only to individuals from a specific group, for example, children, elderly, and obese.

▌ Eating, drinking, dehydration, exercise, and menstrual cycle stage may affect bioimpedance measures. Therefore, client guidelines need to be met to ensure accuracy when using the BIA method.

▌ The BIA method may be more suitable for measuring body composition of obese clients than the SKF method.

Chapter *4*

Near-Infrared Interactance Method

Near-infrared interactance (NIR) is a relatively new field method to estimate body composition. Compared to the skinfold (SKF) and bioelectrical impedance (BIA) methods, which have been validated and refined through years of research, NIR is still in developmental stages. Although NIR has been proposed and marketed as a viable alternative to SKF and BIA methods, much more research is needed to fully evaluate the potential of NIR for body composition assessment.

Near-infrared spectroscopy has been used since 1968 to measure the protein, fat, and water content of agricultural products (Norris, 1983). Conway, Norris, and Bodwell (1984) applied this technology to study human body composition using a high-precision (6 nm), expensive, computerized spectrophotometer. Based on results from a small (N = 17) cross-validation sample, these researchers concluded that this method "successfully predicted % body fat" (p. 1129). However, their NIR prediction equation systematically overestimated relative body fat (%BF) for 10 of the 11 females in the cross-validation sample, indicating that different equations may need to be developed for men and women.

Using computer simulation to predict the accuracy of a low-cost, portable, wide-slit spectrophotometer, Conway and Norris (1987) suggested that a lesser-precision (50 nm instead of 6 nm) instrument, suitable for field work, could be designed. However, the prediction accuracy of the NIR method would be compromised using this device. Shortly thereafter, a less-expensive, commercial NIR analyzer (Futrex-5000) was marketed based on the results of this research (Conway et al., 1984, 1987). The Futrex-5000 analyzer estimates %BF from optical density (OD) measured at only one site. To date, much skepticism surrounds the use of this instrument and the manufacturer's NIR equation to estimate body fatness. Specifically, the following questions have been raised:

1. Is the measurement precision of the Futrex-5000 adequate?
2. Are NIR measures reliable?
3. Is the Futrex-5000 measuring subcutaneous fat only or the tissue composition of the skin, subcutaneous fat, muscle, and possibly even bone at the measurement site?
4. How is total body fat accurately estimated from NIR measurements taken at only one site (the biceps)?
5. Does skin color affect NIR measurements?
6. What are the potential sources of measurement error for this method?
7. How do factors such as age, race, gender, level of body fatness, and physical activity level influence NIR measurements?
8. Is the manufacturer's Futrex-5000 equation valid for estimating %BF? Which population subgroups, if any, can be measured with this equation?
9. Do NIR measurements improve the prediction of body composition compared to using just height and body weight?

Assumptions and Principles of the NIR Method

The near-infrared interactance (NIR) analyzer indirectly measures the tissue composition (fat and water) at various sites. Therefore, certain relationships are assumed when using the NIR method to estimate total body fatness.

Assumptions

1. *The degree of infrared light absorbed and reflected is related both to the composition of the tissues (water, fat, and protein) through which the light is passing and to the specific wavelength of the near-infrared light.* Conway et al. (1984) demonstrated that

a. peak absorption wavelengths for pure fat and pure water are 930 nm and 970 nm, respectively, and
b. the shape of the interactance curve at these two wavelengths is a function of the amount of fat and water present in the sample being measured (Figure 4.1).

The Futrex-5000 measures the OD or the amount of light reflected by the underlying tissues at two wavelengths, 940 nm (OD_1) and 950 nm (OD_2)

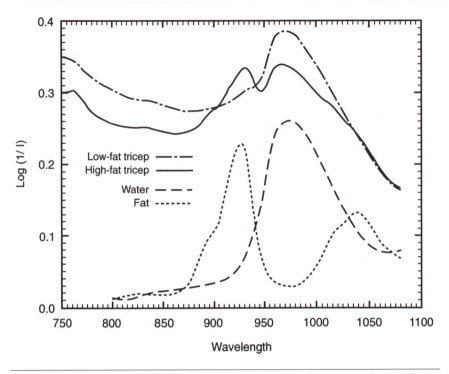

Figure 4.1   Near-infrared spectra for pure fat and distilled water and for low-fat and high-fat triceps sites.

Note. From "A New Approach for the Estimation of Body Composition: Infrared Interactance" by J.M. Conway, K.H. Norris, and C.E. Bodwell, 1984, *American Journal of Clinical Nutrition*, **40**, p. 1125. Copyright 1984 by the *American Journal of Clinical Nutrition*. American Society for Clinical Nutrition. Reprinted with permission.

(Futrex, 1988). It is not clear as to why the manufacturer selected 940 nm and 950 nm wavelengths instead of the 930 nm and 970 nm wavelengths that were identified as the absorption peaks for fat and water. Still, smaller OD measures indicate a greater absorption of the near-infrared light which, in turn, reflects higher fat composition at the measurement site (Conway & Norris, 1987).

   2. *The NIR light penetrates the tissues to a depth of up to 4 cm and is reflected off the bone back to the detector.* Therefore, the OD measures both subcutaneous and intramuscular fat. Although the manufacturer makes this claim, there are no research data to substantiate it. In fact, we found that the slope of the relationship between OD and SKF measures at the biceps site was significantly stronger for leaner women (22 %BF) compared to fatter women (39 %BF) (Quatrochi et al., 1992). This finding suggests that deep penetration (up to 4 cm) of the NIR light beam may be disrupted by fat layering and irregularities at the fat-muscle junction, especially in obese individuals with large amounts of subcutaneous fat.

Principles

1. *Optical densities are linearly related to subcutaneous fat at the biceps site and total body fatness.* The relationship between ODs, subcutaneous fat (skinfold thickness), and %BF depends on the site being measured. Research demonstrates a stronger relationship between OD and SKF measures at the biceps site ($r = -0.66$ to -0.79) compared to other commonly used SKF sites ($r = -0.01$ to -0.48) (Hortobagyi, Israel, Houmard, McCammon, & O'Brien, 1992; McLean & Skinner, 1992; Quatrochi et al., 1992). These findings are surprising given that the biceps site is not commonly found in SKF equations. However, the correlations are only moderate between ODs and SKFs measured at a given site, demonstrating that the OD measure is affected, not only by subcutaneous fat thickness, but also by the composition (fat and water content) of other tissues (skin, muscle, and bone). Conway and Norris (1987) postulated that the combination of skin thickness and subcutaneous fat thickness at the biceps allows sufficient penetration of the near-infrared beam. Thus, the OD at the biceps may be a fairly good indicator of total body fatness (Conway & Norris, 1987).

2. *Age and gender are independent predictors of total body density and %BF.* Data from the first NIR study suggested that the slope and intercept of the regression line depicting the relationship between near-infrared measures and %BF may be different for women and men (Conway et al., 1984). The manufacturer's NIR model includes gender, but not age, as a predictor in the equation. However, some researchers have reported that age is a significant predictor, accounting for an additional 2% to 13% of the variance in total body denisty (Db) (Heyward, Jenkins, et al., 1992; Hicks, Heyward, Flores, et al., 1993; Hortobagyi, Israel, Houmard, O'Brien, et al., 1992). These findings suggest that both age and gender should be included in NIR prediction models, especially if the equations are to be applied to heterogenous populations of males and females varying greatly in age.

NIR Prediction Models

Given that NIR is a relatively new and still unproven method of body composition assessment, there is limited research dealing with the development and testing of NIR prediction models. The manufacturer's NIR model for the Futrex-5000 is a single-site model using ODs at the biceps (OD_1 and OD_2), body weight, height, gender, and exercise level to predict %BF (Futrex, 1988): %BF $= C_0 + C_1(\text{biceps } OD_2) + C_2(\text{gender}) + C_3(\text{body weight in lb}/100) + C_4(\text{height in inches}/100) + C_5(\text{biceps } OD_1) + C_6(\text{exercise level})$. According to the manufacturer, the values of the coefficients, C_0 to C_6, vary among instruments because of small differences in the original optical standard installed in each Futrex-5000 unit (Futrex, 1988).

Researchers have reported that some of the variables in the Futrex-5000 manufacturer's model are not significant predictors of Db and %BF. For example, because there is an extremely strong relationship (r = 0.99) between OD_1 and OD_2 at the biceps site and only a small difference between average OD_1 and OD_2 measurements, only one of these ODs enters the prediction model (Heyward, Jenkins, et al., 1992; Hicks, Heyward, Flores, et al., 1993; Israel et al., 1989). It is important to point out that biceps OD measures (either OD_1 or OD_2) explain a significant proportion (3% to 25%) of the variability in Db or %BF, beyond that accounted for by various combinations of body weight, height, and frame size (Heyward, Jenkins, et al., 1992; Hortobagyi, Israel, Houmard, McCammon, et al., 1992; Hortobagyi, Israel, Houmard, O'Brien, et al., 1992; Houmard et al., 1991; McLean & Skinner, 1992). Also, research confirms that body weight, height, and physical activity level are significant predictors of Db or %BF (Hortabagyi, Israel, Houmard, McCammon, et al., 1992; Israel et al., 1989; McLean & Skinner, 1992). Additionally, age (which is not in the manufacturer's model) should be included in NIR models developed for samples varying greatly in age (Heyward, Jenkins, et al., 1992; Hicks, Heyward, Flores, et al., 1993; Israel et al., 1989; Wilmore, McBride, & Wilmore, 1994).

Although the sum of skinfolds (ΣSKF) from multiple sites is a better indicator of total body fatness than SKF measurements from just one site (Jackson & Pollock, 1985), this is not true for NIR prediction models. As mentioned earlier, the biceps site appears to be the best site for estimating total body fatness with this method. NIR equations using OD measurements from the biceps have smaller prediction errors compared to those using an average or sum of ODs from multiple sites (Conway & Norris, 1987; Elia, Parkinson, & Diaz, 1990; Heyward, Jenkins, et al., 1992; Hortobagyi, Israel, Houmard, McCammon, et al., 1992).

At present there are no NIR equations based on multicomponent model estimates of %BF. However, some NIR equations predict Db (Heyward, Jenkins, et al., 1992; Hicks, Heyward, Flores, et al., 1993) instead of %BF, allowing you to use the appropriate population-specific conversion formula to estimate %BF from Db (Table 1.6).

Using the NIR Method

Because of the limited amount of research in this area, only a few NIR equations can be recommended for various population subgroups (see the Quick Reference Guide in Appendix A). To use these equations, the ODs from the biceps site and the optical standard are measured and recorded. To obtain these values from the Futrex-5000 analyzer, you need to access the OD measurement mode using the following steps (Futrex, 1988):

1. Turn the unit on and let it count down for 15 seconds.
2. Enter "Clear 881." The analyzer will display OD_1.
3. Place the NIR light wand into the optical standard (Teflon block, 1 cm thick). Press "Enter." Your analyzer is programmed by the manufacturer to take two measurements at each site. Therefore, you must press the Enter key twice. OD_1 and OD_2 values for the standard will be alternately displayed. Record these values. The number of measurements taken at the site can be set from one to eight by following the manufacturer's instructions (Futrex, 1988).
4. Place the NIR light probe perpendicular to the measurement site, and press the Enter key the designated number of times (one to eight). OD_1 and OD_2 values for your client will be alternately displayed. Record these values.
5. When assessing many clients during one test session, periodically measure and record the OD values for the optical standard (step #3) every 10 minutes. This corrects for electronic drift in your analyzer (Futrex, 1988).
6. Calculate ΔOD_2 by subtracting the client's OD value from the corresponding standard OD value (e.g., biceps $\Delta OD_2 = OD_2$ standard $- OD_2$ client). Either biceps ΔOD_2 or the $\Sigma \Delta OD_2$ for the pectoral and biceps sites are used in the NIR equations presented in the Quick Reference Guide. The complementary computer software for this book will calculate ΔOD after you enter the standard and client's OD values.

Presently, *we do not recommend using the %BF estimates obtained from your NIR analyzers (Futrex-5000 and Futrex-1000) because numerous researchers have reported unacceptable prediction errors* (SEE = 3.7 %BF to 6.3 %BF) for the Futrex-5000 (Eaton, Israel, O'Brien, Hortobagyi, & McCammon, 1993; Elia et al., 1990; Heyward, Cook, et al., 1992; Heyward, Jenkins, et al., 1992; Hicks, Heyward, Flores, et al., 1993; Hortobagyi, Israel, Houmard, O'Brien, et al., 1992; Houmard et al., 1991; Israel et al., 1989; McLean & Skinner, 1992; Nielsen et al., 1992; Wilson & Heyward, 1993b) and Futrex-1000 (SEE = 4.5 %BF) manufacturer's equations (Belford, Stout, Eckerson, Housh, & Johnson, 1993). The manufacturer's equation systematically underestimated average body fatness by as much as 2 %BF to 10 %BF (Davis, Van Loan, Holly, Krstich, & Phinney, 1989; Elia et al., 1990; Heyward, Cook, et al., 1992; Heyward, Jenkins, et al., 1992; Hicks, Heyward, Flores, et al., 1993; Houmard et al., 1991; Israel et al., 1989). The degree of underestimation of %BF appears to be directly related to the level of body fatness (Elia et al., 1990; Heyward, Cook, et al., 1992). Thus, the %BF of fatter clients is likely to be more grossly underestimated compared to leaner clients when using the Futrex-5000 manufacturer's equation.

Sources of Measurement Error

Research demonstrates high within- and between-day reliability for ODs at the biceps site (r = 0.95 to 0.97) and %BF estimates (r = 0.91 to 0.95) obtained

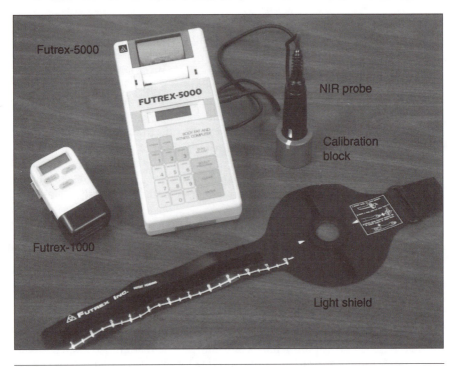

Figure 4.2   Futrex-5000 and Futrex-1000 NIR analyzers.

from the Futrex-5000 (Davis, Dotson, & Manny, 1988; Eaton et al., 1993; Heyward, Jenkins, et al., 1992; Heyward, Jenkins, Mermier, & Stolarczyk, 1993; Hortobagyi, Israel, Houmard, McCammon, et al., 1992). Potential sources of measurement error for the NIR method, such as *instrumentation*, *technician skill*, *subject factors*, and *prediction equations*, have not been adequately identified or studied.

Instrumentation

A highly sophisticated and precise (6 nm) computerized spectrophotometer (Neotec Instruments, Pacific Scientific, Silver Springs, MD) was used to pioneer the application of the NIR method for human body composition assessment and to explore the feasibility of designing a low-cost, less-precise (50 nm) NIR analyzer for this purpose. Apparently, the Futrex-5000 NIR analyzer (Figure 4.2) was developed based on Conway and Norris' (1987) computer-simulated analysis of the expected accuracy for a less expensive, wide-slit (50 nm) spectrophotometer. To our knowledge, OD values from the Futrex-5000 have not been compared to those obtained from the Neotec computerized spectrophotometer. In fact, there is no information available regarding the degree of variation expected when OD measures are taken on the same individual using different Futrex-5000 analyzers.

Futrex also manufactures the Futrex-1000 NIR analyzer (Figure 4.2) which is a hand-held, battery-operated device. This low-cost analyzer supposedly estimates your client's %BF based on OD measurements at the biceps site, body weight and height only. Age and gender are not included. The NIR equation programmed in the Futrex-1000 and research validating its use were not released by the manufacturer when we requested this information. Recently, a large prediction error (SEE = 4.5 %BF) was reported for the Futrex-1000 NIR equation (Belford et al., 1993).

Apparently, a newer version of the NIR analyzer (Futrex-6000) is being developed. However, at present, there is no information available as to how this analyzer and its NIR equations will differ from those of the Futrex-5000.

Technician Skill

Technician skill is not a major source of measurement error for the NIR method. There is little difference in biceps OD values when the same individual is measured independently by two NIR technicians (Heyward et al., 1993). The measurement error associated with differences between technicians was less (2.2% to 2.4%) than that reported (2.8% to 8.8%) for skinfold measures (Lohman, Pollock, et al., 1984; Morrow, Fridye, & Monaghen, 1986). Apparently, the NIR method requires less technician skill than the SKF method because the NIR light probe is placed firmly on the measurement site and does not require isolating the subcutaneous fat from the underlying muscle tissue.

However, the amount of pressure applied to the light probe during measurement may affect OD values. Elia et al. (1990) reported a 10% decrease in OD measurements when pressure applied to the light probe was increased. The manufacturer recommends applying "firm pressure, approximately equal to the pressure of a firm handshake" (Futrex, 1988, p.14). This may be difficult to control among NIR technicians. In addition, the technician should use a light shield (15 cm, doughnut-shaped foam pad) attached to the end of the NIR probe to block out extraneous room light during testing.

Subject Factors

Factors such as skin color and hydration status may be potential sources of error for the NIR method. To date, no one has studied the effects of eating, drinking, exercise, and menstrual cycle stages on OD measurements. We noted that the within-individual variability for biceps OD values measured on different days is 2.1% to 2.4% (Heyward et al., 1993). This source of error was less than that reported for the BIA method (3.1% to 3.9%) (Jackson et al., 1988). With the BIA method, this difference typically reflects changes in total body water (TBW) over test days (Jackson et al., 1988). Assuming that the OD is a measure of the tissue composition (fat and water) at the biceps site, it is feasible that a change in OD values across days may reflect fluctuations in the water content of subcutaneous and muscle tissues. This hypothesis needs to be tested before specific guidelines concerning factors that may potentially affect hydration status, such as eating, drinking, exercising, and testing only at specific stages of the menstrual cycle, can be established.

Skin color or skin tone explains a significant proportion (12% to 16%) of the variability in OD measures at the biceps site, even after controlling for the SKF thickness (Wilson & Heyward, 1993a). We developed a skin-tone wheel and numerically coded various shades of black, brown, red, yellow, pink, and white to assess skintones of a sample of American Indian, black, Hispanic, and white men. The subject's skin color at the biceps site was matched to a color on the skintone wheel. Subjects with darker skintones tended to have higher OD values. Additional research is needed to determine whether or not skintone should be included in NIR prediction models.

NIR Prediction Equations

There are few NIR equations that can be used to accurately assess your client's body fatness. Equations for women (20 to 72 years) and American Indian women (18 to 60 years) have been developed but need further cross-validation (Heyward, Jenkins, et al., 1992; Hicks, Heyward, Flores, et al., 1993). These equations predict Db with a fair (0.0085 g/cc) to good (0.0076 g/cc) degree of accuracy, and they are gender-specific and race-specific. Therefore, these equations cannot be used to accurately estimate body fatness of clients from other population subgroups. Again, we do not recommend using the manufacturer's Futrex-5000 or Futrex-1000 NIR equations because of their large, systematic prediction errors.

NIR Technique

The NIR measurement technique is illustrated in Figure 4.3. Following standardized procedures will increase the accuracy and precision of your OD measurements:

1. Prior to measuring your client, calibrate your analyzer using the optical standard (Teflon block) supplied by the manufacturer. Record the OD_1 and OD_2 standard values.
2. Take NIR measurements on the right side of the body.
3. Carefully identify and mark the NIR site. The biceps OD is measured on the anterior midline over the belly of the biceps brachii muscle, midway between the acromion process of the scapula and the antecubital fossa of the elbow (Futrex, 1988).

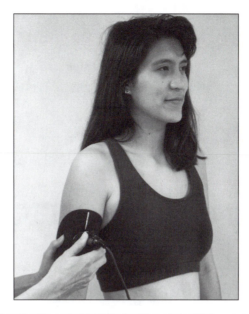

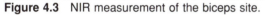

Figure 4.3   NIR measurement of the biceps site.

4. The NIR probe, with its light shield, is firmly placed perpendicular to the measurement site. Use pressure equivalent to a "firm" handshake (Futrex, 1988).
5. Hold the probe firmly in place while your client pushes the Enter key on the analyzer a designated number of times (usually two). Make certain the client uses the left hand when pressing the key pad.
6. Read the digital display which alternately flashes the client's OD_1 and OD_2 values. Record these numbers.

KEY POINTS

▮ The OD is a measure of the fat and water composition of the tissues at the measurement site.
▮ ODs are linearly related to subcutaneous and total body fat.
▮ The biceps is the best single site for estimating body fat using the NIR method.
▮ The manufacturer's NIR equations programmed into the Futrex-1000 and Futrex-5000 analyzers should not be used to estimate your client's level of body fatness.
▮ Much more research is needed to substantiate the validity, accuracy, and applicability of the NIR method for body composition assessment. Therefore, the NIR equations developed for American Indian and white women (see chapter 8) should be used cautiously.

Chapter **5**

Anthropometric Method

Anthropometry refers to the measurement of the size and proportion of the human body. Body weight and stature (standing height) are measures of body size, and ratios of body weight to height can be used to represent body proportion. To assess the size and proportions of body segments, circumferences, skinfold thicknesses, skeletal breadths, and segment lengths may be used.

In addition to measuring body size and proportions, anthropometric measures, like circumferences, skinfolds, and skeletal diameters, have been used to assess total body and regional body composition. Anthropometric indexes, such as body mass index (BMI) and waist-to-hip circumference ratio (WHR) are used to identify individuals at risk for disease. With the exception of skinfold (SKF) measures, anthropometric methods are relatively simple, inexpensive, and do not require a high degree of technicial skill and training. Therefore, these measures are well-suited for large scale, epidemiological surveys and clinical purposes. Although skinfolds are a part of anthropometry, the skinfold method is addressed separately in chapter 2.

Assumptions and Principles of the Anthropometric Method

There are basic principles associated with using anthropometric measures such as BMI, circumferences, and skeletal diameters to estimate body composition:

Assumptions

1. *Circumferences are affected by fat mass, muscle mass, and skeletal size; therefore, these measures are related to fat mass and lean body mass.* Jackson and Pollock (1978) reported that circumference and bony diameter measures are markers of lean body mass (muscle mass and skeletal size); however, some circumferences are also highly associated with the fat component. These findings confirm the fact that circumference measures reflect both the fat and fat-free body components of body composition.

Principles

1. *Skeletal size is directly related to lean body mass.* Behnke (1961) proposed that lean body mass could be accurately estimated from skeletal diameters and developed equations for predicting lean body mass. Cross-validation of these equations yielded a moderately high ($r = 0.80$) relationship and closely estimated the average lean body mass obtained from hydrodensitometry (Wilmore & Behnke, 1969, 1970). Behnke's hypothesis was also supported by the observation that skeletal diameters, along with circumference measures, are strong markers of lean body mass (Jackson & Pollock, 1978).

2. *To estimate total body fat from weight-to-height indexes, the index should be highly related to body fat but independent of height* (Keys, Fidanza, Karvonen, Kimura, & Taylor, 1972; Lee & Hinds, 1981). Based on data from two, large-scale epidemiological surveys (National Health and Nutrition Examination Surveys I and II), Micozzi, Albanes, Jones, and Chumlea (1986) reported that body mass index (body weight divided by height squared) is not significantly related to height of men ($r = -0.06$) and women ($r = -0.16$) but is directly related to skinfold thickness and the estimated fat area of the arm in men and women ($r = 0.72$ to 0.80). However, the relationship to body fat varies with age and gender (Deurenberg, Westrate, & Seidell, 1991). BMI is not totally independent of height, especially in younger children (< 15 years of age). BMI reflects both the lean tissue mass and fat mass of the individual (Garn, Leonard, & Hawthorne, 1986).

Anthropometric Prediction Models

Although some anthropometric prediction models include combinations of skinfolds, circumferences, and skeletal diameters to estimate body composition, only those equations using circumferences and diameters as predictors are addressed in this chapter for the following reasons:

   a. The predictive accuracy of anthropometric (circumference and diameter) equations is not greatly improved by adding skinfold measures.

   b. Anthropometric equations using only circumferences as predictors estimate the body fatness of obese individuals more accurately than skinfold prediction equations (Seip & Weltman, 1991).

   c. Compared to skinfolds, circumferences and skeletal diameters can be measured with less error (Bray & Gray, 1988a).

   d. Some practitioners may not have access to skinfold calipers.

Anthropometric prediction equations estimate total body density (Db), relative body fat (%BF), or fat-free mass (FFM) from combinations of body weight, height, skeletal diameters, and circumference measures. Generally, equations with only skeletal measures as predictors have larger prediction errors than those using both circumferences and bony diameters as predictors (Boileau, Wilmore, Lohman, Slaughter, & Riner, 1981; Katch & McArdle, 1973). Like SKF and bioelectrical impedance (BIA) equations, anthropometric equations are based on either population-specific or generalized models.

Population-specific anthropometric equations are valid for and can only be applied to individuals whose physical characteristics (age, gender, and level of body fatness) are similar to those in a specific population subgroup. For example, anthropometric equations developed to estimate the body composition of obese individuals (Weltman, Levine, Seip, & Tran, 1988; Weltman, Seip, & Tran, 1987) should not be applied to nonobese individuals.

On the other hand, generalized equations, applicable to individuals varying in age and body fatness, have been developed for heterogenous populations of women (15 to 79 years of age; 13 %BF to 63 %BF) and men (20 to 78 years of age; 2 %BF to 49 %BF) (Tran & Weltman, 1988, 1989). The predictive accuracy of these generalized equations for estimating %BF of obese men and women was similar to that of fatness-specific (obese) equations (Seip & Weltman, 1991). Typically, generalized equations include body weight or height, along with two or three circumferences, as predictors of Db or %BF. Like generalized SKF models, the relationship between some circumference measures and Db is curvilinear (Tran & Weltman, 1988, 1989). Also, age was an independent predictor of Db for women (Tran & Weltman, 1989).

Although BMI is related to fat mass and %BF (r = 0.75 to 0.98), the prediction errors are generally large (SEE = 3.8 %BF to 5.8 %BF) when BMI is used as a single predictor of body fatness (Deurenberg, Westrate, & Seidell, 1991; Garrow & Webster, 1985; Gray & Fujioka, 1991; Jackson et al., 1988; Smalley, Knerr, Kendrick, Colliver, & Owens, 1990; Strain & Zumoff, 1992). Two reasons why BMI is limited in its ability to predict %BF and to accurately classify levels of body fatness (Lohman, 1992) are:

   1. Individuals with a large musculoskeletal system in relation to their height can have BMI values in the obese range even though they are

not overly fat. Conversely, those with relatively small musculoskeletal systems tend to have lower BMI values.

2. BMI does not detect or reflect differential growth rates of muscle and bone in children or differential rates of muscle and bone loss in older individuals.

Using the Anthropometric Method

Anthropometric prediction equations that are applicable to various population subgroups are presented in chapters 6 to 10 and summarized in the Quick Reference Guide in Appendix A. You can use the complementary computer software to obtain body composition estimates from these equations for your clients.

Sources of Measurement Error

The accuracy and reliability of anthropometric measures can be affected by *equipment, technician skill, subject factors, and the prediction equation selected to estimate body composition* (Bray et al., 1978; Callaway et al., 1988). As with other body composition methods, the total prediction error is a function of the errors associated with both the anthropometric method and the reference method used to develop the prediction equation. Acceptable errors for estimating relative body fatness (%BF) and fat-free mass (FFM) are $\leq 3.5\ \%BF$ and $\leq 2.8\ kg$ (for women) and $\leq 3.5\ kg$ (for men), respectively (Table 1.8).

Equipment

Skeletal anthropometers and sliding or spreading calipers are used to measure bony widths and body breadths (Figure 5.1). The precision characteristic (0.05 cm to 0.50 cm) and range of measurement (0 to 210 cm) depends on the type of skeletal anthropometer or caliper you are using (Wilmore et al., 1988). The instruments need to be carefully maintained and calibrated periodically to check their accuracy.

Use an anthropometric tape measure to measure circumferences (Figure 5.1). The tape measure should be made from a flexible material that does not stretch with use. Plastic-coated tape measures can be used if an anthropometric tape measure is not available. Some anthropometric tapes have a spring-loaded handle (Gulick handle) that allows a constant tension to be applied to the end of the tape during the measurement. Use of the

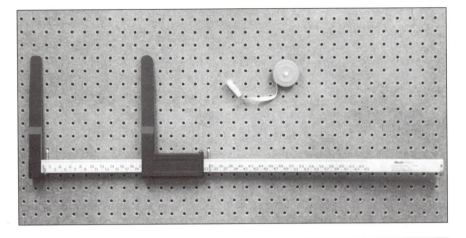

Figure 5.1   Broad-blade skeletal anthropometer and anthropometric tape measure.

spring-loaded handle is not recommended for circumference measurements requiring minimal tension (e.g., neck circumference) (Callaway et al., 1988).

Technician Skill

Compared to the SKF method, *technician skill is not a major source of measurement error, provided that standardized procedures are closely followed for locating measurement sites, positioning of the anthropometer or tape measure, and applying tension during the measurement.* Some of the most commonly used circumference and skeletal diameter sites are described in Tables 5.1 and 5.2 and illustrated in Figures 5.2 and 5.3.

Variability in circumference measurements taken by different technicians is relatively small (0.2 cm to 1.0 cm), with some sites differing more than others (Callaway et al., 1988). Skilled technicians can obtain similar values, even when measuring circumferences of obese individuals (Bray et al., 1978). However, practice is needed to perfect the identification of the measurement site and your measurement technique. *Some experts recommend practicing on at least 50 people and taking a minimum of three measurements for each site in rotational order* (Callaway et al., 1988; Katch & Katch, 1980).

Subject Factors

Accurate measurement of bony diameters in heavily-muscled or obese individuals may be difficult because the underlying muscle and fat tissues

Table 5.1   Standardized Sites for Circumference Measurements

Site	Anatomical reference	Position	Measurement
Neck	Laryngeal prominence—Adam's apple	Perpendicular to long axis of neck	Apply tape with minimal pressure just inferior to the Adam's apple.
Shoulder	Deltoid muscles and acromion processes of scapula	Horizontal	Apply tape snugly over maximum bulges of the deltoid muscles, inferior to acromion processes. Record measurement at end of normal expiration.
Chest	Fourth costo-sternal joints	Horizontal	Apply tape snugly around the torso at level of fourth costo-sternal joints. Record at end of normal expiration.
Waist	Narrowest part of torso, level of the "natural" waist between ribs and iliac crest	Horizontal	Apply tape snugly around the waist at level of narrowest part of torso. An assistant is needed to position tape behind the client. Take measurement at end of normal expiration.
Abdominal	Maximum anterior protuberance of abdomen, usually at umbilicus	Horizontal	Apply tape snugly around the abdomen at level of greatest anterior protuberance. An assistant is needed to position tape behind the client. Take measurement at end of normal expiration.
Hip (buttocks)	Maximum posterior extension of buttocks	Horizontal	Apply tape snugly around the buttocks. An assistant is needed to position tape on opposite side of body.
Thigh *Proximal*	Gluteal fold	Horizontal	Apply tape snugly around thigh, just distal to the gluteal fold.
Mid	Inguinal crease and proximal border of patella	Horizontal	With client's knee flexed 90° (right foot on bench), apply tape at level midway between inguinal crease and proximal border of patella.

(continued)

Table 5.1 *(continued)*

Site	Anatomical reference	Position	Measurement
Thigh *(continued)*			
Distal	Femoral epicondyles	Horizontal	Apply tape just proximal to the femoral epicondyles.
Knee	Patella	Horizontal	Apply tape around the knee at mid-patellar level with knee relaxed in slight flexion.
Calf	Maximum girth of calf muscle	Perpendicular to long axis of leg	With client sitting on end of table, and legs hanging freely, apply tape horizontally around the maximum girth of calf.
Ankle	Malleoli of tibia and fibula	Perpendicular to long axis of leg	Apply tape snugly around minimum circumference of leg, just proximal to the malleoli.
Arm (biceps)	Acromion process of scapula and olecranon process of ulna	Perpendicular to long axis of arm	With arms hanging freely at sides and palms facing thighs, apply tape snugly around the arm at level midway between the acromion process of scapula and olecranon process of ulna (as marked for triceps and biceps SKFs).
Forearm	Maximum girth of forearm	Perpendicular to long axis of forearm	With arms hanging down and away from trunk and forearm supinated, apply tape snugly around the maximum girth of the proximal part of the forearm.
Wrist	Styloid processes of radius and ulna	Perpendicular to long axis of forearm	With elbow flexed and forearm supinated, apply tape snugly around wrist, just distal to the styloid processes of the radius and ulna.

Note. Adapted from Callaway et al. (1988, pp. 41-53.).

Table 5.2   Standardized Sites for Bony Breadth Measurements

Site	Anatomical reference	Position	Measurement
Biacromial (shoulder)	Lateral borders of acromion processes of scapula	Horizontal	With client standing, arms hanging vertically and shoulders relaxed, downward and slightly forward, apply blades of anthropometer to lateral borders of acromion processes. Measurement is taken from the rear.
Chest	Sixth ribs on mid-axillary line or fourth costo-sternal joints anteriorly	Horizontal	With client standing, arms slightly abducted, apply the large spreading caliper tips lightly on the sixth ribs on the midaxillary line. Take measurement at end of normal expiration.
Bi-iliac (bicristal)	Iliac crests	45° downward angle	With client standing, arms folded across the chest, apply anthropometer blades firmly at a 45° downward angle, at maximum breadth of iliac crest. Measurement is taken from rear.
Bitrochanteric	Greater trochanter of femur	Horizontal	With client standing, arms folded across the chest, apply anthropometer blade with considerable pressure to compress soft tissues. Measure maximum distance between the trochanters from the rear.
Knee	Femoral epicondyles	Diagonal or horizontal	With client sitting and knee flexed to 90°, apply caliper blades firmly on lateral and medial femoral epicondyles.

(continued)

Table 5.2   *(continued)*

Site	Anatomical reference	Position	Measurement
Ankle (bimalleolar)	Malleoli of tibia and fibula	Oblique	With client standing and weight evenly distributed, place the caliper blades on the most lateral part of lateral malleolus and most medial part of medial malleolus. Measurement is taken on an oblique plane from the rear.
Elbow	Epicondyles of humerus	Oblique	With elbow flexed 90°, arm raised to the horizontal, and forearm supinated, apply the caliper blades firmly to the medial and lateral humeral epicondyles at an angle that bisects the right angle at the elbow.
Wrist	Styloid process of radius and ulna, anatomical "snuff box"	Oblique	With elbow flexed 90°, upper arm vertical and close to torso, and forearm pronated, apply caliper tips firmly at an oblique angle to the styloid processes of the radius (at proximal part of anatomical snuff box) and ulna.

Note. Adapted from Wilmore et al. (1988, pp. 28-38).

must be firmly compressed. Bony anatomical landmarks may not be readily identified and palpated, leading to error in locating the measurement site.

Like the SKF method, it is more difficult to obtain consistent measurements of circumference for obese compared to lean individuals (Bray & Gray, 1988a). However, circumferences are preferable to SKFs when measuring obese clients for these reasons:

a. Regardless of their size, circumferences of obese individuals can be measured; whereas the maximum aperature of the SKF caliper may not be large enough to allow measurement.

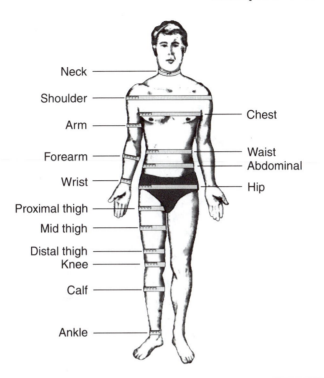

Figure 5.2 Anatomical sites for circumferences.

---

b. Circumferences require less technician skill, and the difference between technicians is smaller compared to SKF measurements (Bray & Gray, 1988a).

In addition, you should be aware of the possibility that the accuracy of circumference measurements may be affected by fluid retention and subcutaneous edema, particularly in women experiencing large weight gains during certain stages of their menstrual cycle.

Anthropometric Prediction Equations

As mentioned earlier, anthropometric prediction equations should be selected based on the gender, age, and level of body fatness of your client. Using an inappropriate equation may produce systematic prediction error in estimating body composition. *We do not recommend using BMI to estimate body fatness of your clients because of the large prediction error associated with this method.*

Finally, we would like to comment on the accuracy and use of anthropometric prediction equations developed to assess and monitor body fat

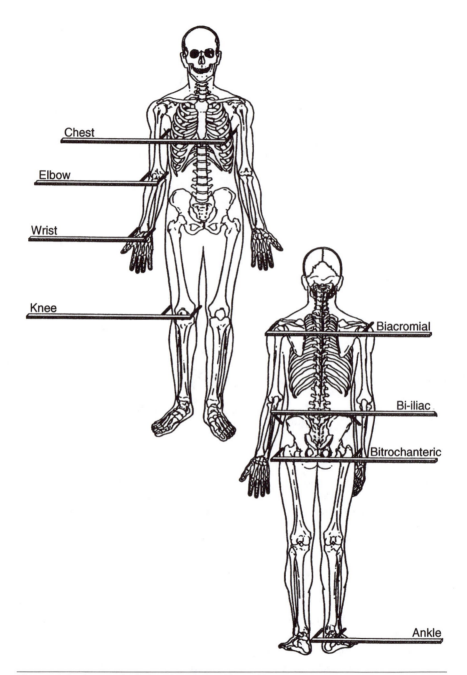

Figure 5.3 Anatomical sites for skeletal breadth measures.

levels of military personnel in the United States. These equations use various combinations of body weight, height, neck, abdomen, hip, thigh, arm, forearm, and wrist circumferences to predict either FFM or %BF. Cross-validation of each equation developed for men and women in the Army, Navy, Air Force, and Marines yielded large, unacceptable prediction errors (SEE = 3.7 %BF to 5.2 %BF) (Hodgdon, 1992). Therefore, the practice of dismissing personnel from the armed services because their %BF exceeds military standards may be questionable when their %BF is estimated from these anthropometric equations. Instead, *technicians should consider using a reference method, like hydrodensitometry, instead of field methods to assess body composition of military personnel facing this problem.*

Anthropometric Techniques

Practice is necessary to become proficient in measuring skeletal diameters and circumferences. Following standardized procedures will increase the accuracy and reliability of your measurements (Callaway et al., 1988; Wilmore et al., 1988).

Cirumferences and Skeletal Diameters

1. Take all circumference and bony diameter measurements of the limbs on the right side of the body.
2. Carefully identify and measure the anthropometric site. Be meticulous about locating anatomical landmarks used to identify the measurement site.
3. Take a minimum of three measurements at each site in rotational order.
4. Small sliding calipers (a range of 30 cm) with greater scale precision should be used instead of larger skeletal anthropometers (a range of 60 cm to 80 cm) to measure the breadth of smaller segments, like the elbow and wrist.
5. The skeletal anthropometer or caliper is held in both hands so the tips of the index fingers are adjacent to the tips of the caliper.
6. The caliper is placed on the bony landmarks and firm pressure is applied to compress the underlying muscle, fat, and skin. Apply pressure to a point where the measurement no longer continues to decrease.
7. Use an anthropometric tape to measure circumferences. The zero end of the tape is held in your left hand and is positioned below the other part of the tape held in your right hand.

8. Tension should be applied to the tape so that it fits snugly around the body part but does not indent the skin or compress the subcutaneous tissue.
9. For some circumferences (e.g., waist, hip, and thigh), the tape should be aligned in a horizontal plane, parallel to the floor.

In addition, standardized procedures for measuring body weight and stature (standing height), as recommended in the *Anthropometric Standardization Reference Manual* (Gordon, Chumlea, & Roche, 1988), should be followed.

Body Weight

1. A beam scale with moveable weights or an electronic digital scale is used to measure body weight to the nearest 100 g. Spring scales are not recommended.
2. To measure body weight, the subject stands on the platform of the scale with the body weight evenly distributed between the feet. Light, indoor clothing (but no shoes) may be worn; however, a disposable paper gown is preferred to standardize this measure. One trial is usually sufficient to obtain an accurate measurement of body weight.
3. The accuracy of the scale should be checked periodically by placing standard calibration weights (Toledo Scale, Toledo, OH) on the scale. If the scale weight does not match the calibration weight, balance the scale by adjusting its calibration screw while the calibration weight is on the scale.

Stature (Standing Height)

1. A stadiometer with a fixed or moveable rod is used to measure standing height. Stature may be measured against a wall, if the wall does not have a baseboard and the floor is not carpeted.
2. The client is barefoot and stands on a flat surface that is at a right angle to the vertical rod or board of the stadiometer. The weight is evenly distributed between both feet, and the arms are hanging by the sides with palms facing the thighs. The heels are together, touching the vertical board of the stadiometer. The feet are spread at a 60° angle to each other. Whenever possible, the head, scapula, and buttocks should also be touching the vertical board. The head is erect with eyes focused straight ahead.
3. As the client inhales deeply, the horizontal board of the stadiometer is lowered to the most superior point on the head, compressing the hair. Standing height is measured to the nearest 0.1 cm.

Body Mass Index (BMI)

BMI is the ratio of body weight to height squared: BMI (kg/m^2) = WT (in kg)/HT^2 (in m). To calculate BMI, the body weight is measured in kilograms and the height is converted from centimeters to meters (cm/100). Alternatively, a nomogram (Figure 5.4) can be used to calculate and classify your client's BMI (Bray, 1978). You should be aware that the versions of Bray's nomogram appearing in *The Surgeon General's Report on Nurition and Health* (U.S. Department of Health and Human Services, 1988) and *Diet and Health* (National Research Council, 1989) are inaccurate because the orientation of the vertical columns of the original nomogram was mistakenly altered by the graphic artist (Kahn, 1991).

Standards for classifying BMI are presented in Table 5.3. It is important to remember that BMI is only a crude index of obesity and should not be used to estimate body fatness of your clients.

Anthropometric Indexes of Body Fat Distribution

Research indicates that the way in which fat is distributed in the body is more important than total body fat for determining one's risk of disease (Ashwell, McCall, Cole, & Dixon, 1985). Vague (1947) introduced a system for differentiating types of obesity based on regional fat distribution. He coined the terms "android obesity" and "gynoid obesity" to describe individuals who localize excess body fat mainly in the upper body (android) or lower body (gynoid). Android obesity is more typical of males; gynoid obesity is more characteristic of females. However, obese men and women can be, and often are, classified into either group. There are other terms used to describe types of obesity and regional fat distribution. Android obesity (apple-shaped) is frequently referred to as upper-body obesity, and gynoid obesity (pear-shaped) is often described as lower-body obesity.

The impact of regional fat distribution on health is related to the amount of visceral fat located within the abdominal cavity. The proliferation of research on body fat distribution and its relationship to disease has expanded at an exponential rate over the past 10 years, providing clear evidence that a link exists between increased abdominal fat and increased morbidity and mortality (Despres, 1991). This research demonstrates strong associations between abdominal fat and diseases such as coronary artery disease (Donahue, Abbot, Bloom, Reed, & Yano, 1987; Ducimetier, Richard, & Cambien, 1989; Larsson et al., 1984), diabetes (Bjorntorp, 1988), hypertension (Blair, Habricht, Sims, Sylwester, & Abraham, 1984; White, Periera, & Garner, 1986), and hyperlipidemia (Blair et al., 1984; Despres, Fong, Julien, Jimenez, & Angel, 1987).

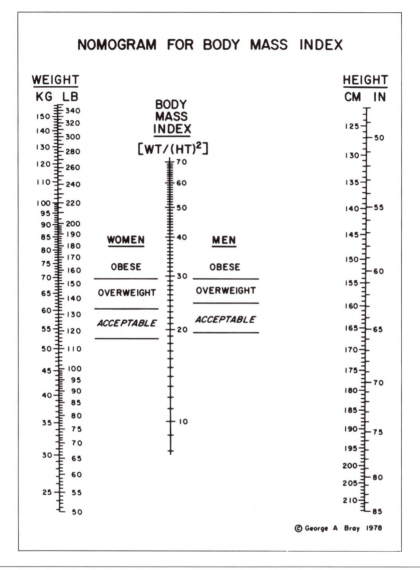

Figure 5.4 Nomogram for body mass index (BMI).

Note. From "Definitions, Measurements and Classifications of the Syndromes of Obesity" by G.A. Bray, 1978, *International Journal of Obesity*, **2**(2). Copyright 1978 by G.A. Bray. Reprinted with permission.

Table 5.3   Obesity Classification Based on Body Mass Index (BMI)

Classification	Men	Women
Normal	24-27	23-26
Moderately obese	28-31	27-32
Severely obese	> 31	> 32

Note. Data from *The Surgeon General's Report on Nutrition and Health* (U.S. Department of Health and Human Services, 1988 p. 284).

Anthropometric indexes can be used to classify individuals according to their type of obesity, such as upper-body or abdominal obesity (high-risk) or lower-body obesity (low-risk). Numerous anthropometric measures are significantly related to intra-abdominal fat: skinfold measures of the trunk (umbilicus, suprailiac, and subscapular), waist and hip circumferences, the ratio of the waist-to-hip circumference (WHR), sagittal diameter, body mass index (BMI), and age (Despres, Prud'homme, Pouliot, Tremblay, & Bouchard, 1991; Ferland et al., 1989; Seidell et al., 1987, 1989; Svendsen, Hassager, Bergmann, & Christiansen, 1992; Weits, Van der Beek, Wedel, & Ter Haar Romeny, 1988; Zamboni et al., 1992). There are only two anthropometric indexes, BMI and WHR, that are widely recognized for their ability to predict disease risk. These two indexes have established norms and standards for classifying individuals into high- or low-risk categories.

Waist-To-Hip Ratio

Waist-to-hip ratio (WHR) is strongly associated with visceral fat (Ashwell et al., 1985; Seidell et al., 1987) and appears to be an acceptable index of intra-abdominal fat (Jakicic, 1993). However, some researchers (Despres et al., 1991; Weits et al., 1988) found waist circumference alone to be a better predictor of visceral fat deposition than WHR. This finding supports the hypothesis that abdominal fat deposition could increase waist circumference regardless of whether adipose tissue accumulates in deep or superficial sites (Busetto et al., 1992). Hip circumference, however, is influenced by subcutaneous fat deposition only; thus, the accuracy of WHR in assessing visceral fat decreases with increasing levels of fatness. WHR can change depending on the menopausal status of women (Weits et al., 1988; Svendsen et al., 1992). Postmenopausal women show more of a male pattern of fat distribution than premenopausal women (Ferland et al., 1989).

Despite these discrepancies, no norms have been established for waist circumference. Therefore, we recommend that you classify clients into

Table 5.4   Waist-To-Hip Circumference Ratio (WHR) Norms for Men and Women

			Risk		
	Age	Low	Moderate	High	Very high
Men	20-29	< 0.83	0.83-0.88	0.89-0.94	> 0.94
	30-39	< 0.84	0.84-0.91	0.92-0.96	> 0.96
	40-49	< 0.88	0.88-0.95	0.96-1.00	> 1.00
	50-59	< 0.90	0.90-0.96	0.97-1.02	> 1.02
	60-69	< 0.91	0.91-0.98	0.99-1.03	> 1.03
Women	20-29	< 0.71	0.71-0.77	0.78-0.82	> 0.82
	30-39	< 0.72	0.72-0.78	0.79-0.84	> 0.84
	40-49	< 0.73	0.73-0.79	0.80-0.87	> 0.87
	50-59	< 0.74	0.74-0.81	0.82-0.88	> 0.88
	60-69	< 0.76	0.76-0.83	0.84-0.90	> 0.90

Note. Adapted from Bray and Gray (1988b, p. 432).

low- or high-risk categories using the WHR. Generally, young adults with WHR values in excess of 0.94 for men and 0.82 for women are at high risk for adverse health consequences (Bray & Gray, 1988b). However, this index is not valid for evaluating fat distribution in prepubertal children (Peters, Fox, Armstrong, Sharpe, & Bell, 1992). Also, WHR cannot be used to accurately predict changes in visceral fat (van der Kooy et al., 1993).

The procedures for measuring waist and hip circumferences have not been universally standardized. The World Health Organization (1988) recommends measuring waist circumference midway between the lower rib margin and the iliac crest and hip circumference at the widest point over the greater trochanters. In contrast, the *Anthropometric Standardization Reference Manual* (Callaway et al., 1988) recommends measuring the waist circumference at the narrowest part of the torso and hip circumference at the level of the maximum extension of the buttocks (Figure 5.5a-b). The WHR norms (Table 5.4) were established using the standardized measurement procedures described in the *Anthropometric Standardization Reference Manual*. The WHR is simply calculated by dividing waist circumference (measured in cm) by hip circumference (measured in cm). Alternatively, a nomogram (Figure 5.6) can be used to obtain WHR.

Conicity Index

The conicity index (C-index) is another anthropometric measure having potential for predicting fat distribution and disease risk (Valdez, 1991). *The*

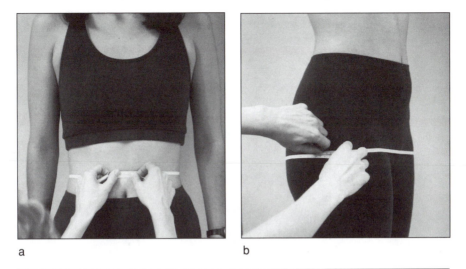

Figure 5.5 Measurement of the (a) waist and (b) hip circumferences.

C-index is based upon the idea that the shape of the human body changes from that of a cylinder to that of a "double cone" with the accumulation of fat around the waist (Figure 5.7). The C-index is calculated using the following equation: C-index = Waist C/0.109 $\sqrt{(WT/HT)}$, where Waist C is waist circumference (m), WT is body weight (kg), and HT is height (m). The theoretical range for the C-index is 1.00 (perfect cylinder) to 1.73 (perfect double cone).

In a large-scale epidemiological study that included seven populations of men and women from Europe and the United States, Valdez, Seidell, Ahn, and Weiss (1992) compared the relationship between WHR and the C-index with several health indicators (total cholesterol, high-density lipoprotein, low-density lipoprotein, triglycerides, and insulin). The relationships of these parameters to WHR and C-index were similar ($r = 0.45$ to 0.86) for the different populations.

We further examined the utility of this index in a large sample of American Indian women and found that the C-index and WHR were highly correlated ($r = 0.88$). The relationship of C-index and WHR to trunk fat, assessed by dual-energy x-ray absorptiometry, was similar ($r = 0.56$ and 0.50, respectively).

Although further investigation is needed to determine the viability of using the C-index to predict abdominal adiposity and concomitant health risk, it has several advantages over WHR:

a. It has an expected theoretical range (1.0 to 1.73).
b. It compares the individual's waist circumference to the circumference of a perfect cyclinder with the same body volume, thereby providing a relative measure of abdominal obesity.
c. The C-indexes of individuals who differ in body weight and height can be compared.

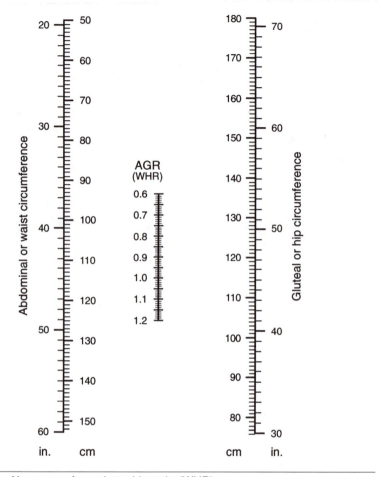

Figure 5.6   Nomogram for waist-to-hip ratio (WHR).
Note. From "Obesity: Part I—Pathogenesis" by G.A. Bray and D.S. Gray, 1988b, *Western Journal of Medicine,* **149**, p. 432. Copyright 1988 by *The Western Journal of Medicine.* Reprinted with permission.

d. It does not require measurement of hip circumference (Valdez et al., 1992). However, until norms are established for this index, the C-index has limited applicability in clinical settings.

Additional Applications of Anthropometry

Various combinations of skinfold, circumference, and skeletal diameter measures can be used to assess your client's body profile (somatogram) and to classify frame size.

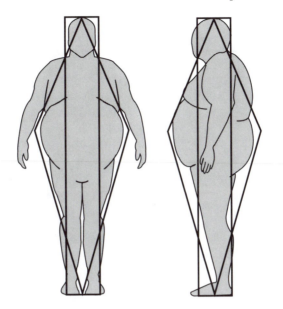

Figure 5.7 Double cone vs. perfect cylinder models to depict shape of human body with increased abdominal adiposity.
Note. From "A New Index of Abdominal Adiposity as an Indicator of Risk for Cardiovascular Disease. A Cross-Population Study" by R. Valdez, J.C. Seidell, Y.I. Ahn, and K.M. Weiss, 1992, *International Journal of Obesity*, **17**, p. 78. Copyright 1992 by MacMillan Press, Ltd. Reprinted with permission.

Somatogram

A somatogram is an anthropometric profile that graphically depicts your client's pattern of muscle and fat distribution (Figure 5.8). Circumferences for six muscular components (shoulders, chest, arm, forearm, thigh, and calf) and five nonmuscular components (umbilicus, hip, knee, wrist, and ankle) are measured. The relative deviation (%) of each circumference measurement from its reference value is calculated and graphed to visually display the individual's body profile. Somatograms may be especially useful for charting changes (pre- and post-test profiles) and monitoring progress of clients involved in weight management (diet and exercise) programs. To assess your client's body profile, use the following steps:

1. Measure the 11 circumferences, as described in Table 5.1, to the nearest 0.1 cm using an anthropometric measuring tape. Measure the thigh circumference at the proximal location.
2. The reference value (R) is calculated by summing the 11 circumferences and dividing by 100, which is the sum of the constant (k) values for the reference body (see Table 5.5): R = Σ11 circumferences/100.

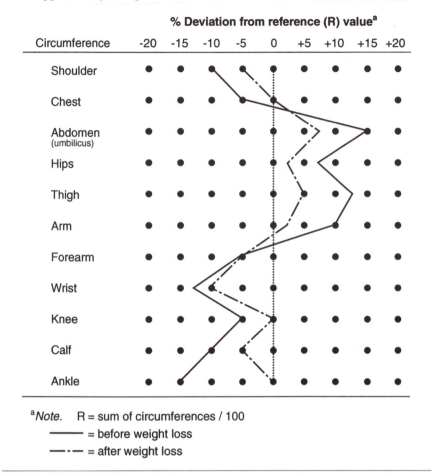

Figure 5.8 Anthropometric profile (somatogram) of a 45-year-old woman before and after weight loss.

3. Divide each circumference by its corresponding k value (Table 5.5) to obtain the d value: d = C/k.
4. Subtract the reference value (R) obtained in step 2 from each d value calculated in step 3 to obtain the absolute difference (AD) score: AD = d-R. Note that when R is greater than d, a negative AD value will be obtained.
5. Calculate the relative difference (%) by dividing each AD score by the R value: % = AD/R.
6. Plot the % obtained for each circumference on a blank somatogram.

Frame Size

Skeletal diameters can be used to classify frame size in order to improve the validity of using height-weight tables for evaluating body weight of

Table 5.5 Somatogram Constants (k) for a Reference Man and Woman

Circumference	Reference man	Reference woman
Shoulder	18.47	17.51
Chest	15.30	14.85
Abdomen	13.07	12.90
Hips	15.57	16.93
Thigh	9.13	10.03
Arm	5.29	4.80
Forearm	4.47	4.15
Wrist	2.88	2.73
Knee	6.10	6.27
Calf	5.97	6.13
Ankle	3.75	3.70
	100.00	100.00

Note. Reference man and woman, ages 20-24 years (Behnke & Wilmore, 1974).

your client. The rationale for including frame size is that skeletal breadths are important estimators of the bone and muscle components of FFM. Therefore, an estimate of frame size allows you to differentiate between those who weigh more because of a large musculoskeletal mass and those who are overweight because of a large fat mass (Himes & Frisancho, 1988). Because there are health implications for individuals who are overweight, critical evaluation of body weight is important.

There are numerous skeletal measurements that can be used to estimate frame size; however, the best estimators of frame size for evaluating body weight are those that are highly related to FFM (independent of stature) and poorly related to fat mass. Himes and Bouchard (1985) noted that wrist and ankle breadths are the best indicators of frame size. Unfortunately, there are no reference norms for these measures. Frisancho and Flegel (1983) reported that elbow breadth is a good predictor of frame size because of its weak association with skinfold (triceps and subscapular) measures. Given that reference data are available for elbow breadth, this measure can be used to classify your client's frame size (Table 5.6). The anatomical landmarks for measuring elbow breadth are described in Table 5.2.

Table 5.6   Elbow Breadth Norms for Men and Women in the United States

	Age (years)	Frame size		
		Small	Medium	Large
Men	18-24	≤ 6.6	> 6.6 and < 7.7	≥ 7.7
	25-34	≤ 6.7	> 6.7 and < 7.9	≥ 7.9
	35-44	≤ 6.7	> 6.7 and < 8.0	≥ 8.0
	45-54	≤ 6.7	> 6.7 and < 8.1	≥ 8.1
	55-64	≤ 6.7	> 6.7 and < 8.1	≥ 8.1
	65-74	≤ 6.7	> 6.7 and < 8.1	≥ 8.1
Women	18-24	≤ 5.6	> 5.6 and < 6.5	≥ 6.5
	25-34	≤ 5.7	> 5.7 and < 6.8	≥ 6.8
	35-44	≤ 5.7	> 5.7 and < 7.1	≥ 7.1
	45-54	≤ 5.7	> 5.7 and < 7.2	≥ 7.2
	55-64	≤ 5.8	> 5.8 and < 7.2	≥ 7.2
	65-74	≤ 5.8	> 5.8 and < 7.2	≥ 7.2

Note. From "New Standard of Weight and Body Composition by Frame Size and Height for Assessment of Nutritional Status of Adults and the Elderly" by A.R. Frisancho, 1984, *American Journal of Clinical Nutrition*, **40**, p. 810. Copyright 1984 by the American Journal of Clinical Nutrition of the American Society for Clinical Nutrition. Reprinted with permission.

KEY POINTS

▮ Circumference measures are affected by fat, muscle mass, and skeletal size. Skeletal size is directly related to lean body mass.

▮ Anthropometric prediction equations include combinations of various circumferences and bony diameter measures and are based on either population-specific or generalized models.

▮ Anthropometric prediction equations are better than skinfold equations for estimating body composition of obese individuals.

▮ BMI is a crude index of overall body fatness and, therefore, should not be used to classify your client's level of body fatness.

▮ Intra-abdominal fat may be a better predictor of disease risk than total body fat. WHR is an acceptable index of intra-abdominal fat.

▮ A somatogram is an anthropometric profile depicting the regional distribution of fat and muscle in the body.

Part II

Body Composition Methods and Equations for Specific Populations

Chapter 6

Body Composition and Children

In chapter 1, the limitations of using the two-component model to estimate relative body fatness of individuals whose fat-free body (FFB) composition differs from the assumed constants (73.8% water, 19.4% protein, and 6.8% mineral) were addressed. The two-component model is especially limited in children because of changes in the proportions and densities of the FFB components due to growth and maturation. These changes in the density of the FFB in children are due to the decreases in total body water and increases in bone mineral during growth and development. Therefore, prediction equations based on the two-component models of Siri (1961) and Brozek et al. (1963) tend to systematically overestimate the relative body fat (%BF) in children by 2% to 4% (Lohman, 1992; Nielsen et al., 1993). Experts recommend using a multicomponent body composition model to establish reference data and to develop prediction equations for children (Lohman, 1992).

To assess the body composition of children, the skinfold (SKF) or bioelectrical impedance (BIA) methods can be used. Selected SKF and BIA equations for children are presented in Table 6.1 and in the Quick Reference Guide in Appendix A.

In this chapter, prediction equations for assessing body composition of children were selected using the criteria outlined in chapter 1, with the following modifications:

1. The prediction error (standard error of estimate or SEE) for estimating fat-free mass (FFM) of children should be less (2.2 kg) than the maximum values (SEE = 2.8 kg for women and 3.5 kg for men) for adults because of the relatively smaller FFM in children.

2. Whenever possible, the selected prediction equations were derived from either (a) multicomponent models that account for interindividual variability in the water and mineral components of the FFB, or (b) two-component model conversion formulas that adjust for changes in the density of the FFB.

3. Although some prediction equations use combinations of variables from different body composition methods (e.g., skinfold, bioelectrical impedance, and circumferences) in the same equation, the improvement in the predictive accuracy of these equations is not large enough to warrant their inclusion (Guo et al., 1989; Houtkooper, Lohman, Going, & Hall, 1989; Houtkooper, Going, Lohman, Roche, & Van Loan, 1992). These equations may not be practical in clinical or school settings because the practitioner needs to have a bioelectrical impedance analyzer, skinfold caliper, and anthropometric tape measure to measure all of these variables. Therefore, whenever possible, we selected only "pure" prediction equations for each field method (i.e., skinfold measures only for SKF equations, bioimpedance measures only for BIA equations, optical density measures only for NIR equations, and circumference and skeletal breadth measures only for anthropometric equations).

Assessing Body Composition of Children

Body composition measures can be used to monitor changes during growth and development and to classify the level of body fatness in children. Research shows that fatter children have a stronger tendency to be obese as adults (Abraham & Nordsieck, 1960; Charney, Goodman, McBridge, Lyon, & Pratt, 1976) and a relatively greater health risk for cardiovascular disease (Williams, Going, Lohman, Harsha, et al., 1992). Boys with > 25% relative body fat and girls with > 30% relative body fat have higher systolic and diastolic blood pressures, total cholesterol, and lipoprotein cholesterol ratios (the ratio of LDL-cholesterol to HDL-cholesterol), indicating a greater relative risk for developing cardiovascular disease (Williams, Going, Lohman, Harsha, et al., 1992).

In school settings, health and physical educators need to interpret body composition results for children and parents. Children should be taught how to achieve and maintain healthy body fat levels through lifestyle modifications (e.g., physical activity and nutrition). Information about changes in body composition and body fatness due to maturation should be addressed so that the children, especially girls, can understand that these changes in their bodies during puberty are normal. Based on work by Thomas and Whitehead (1993), we suggest the following approach for incorporating body composition into the health and physical education curriculum:

1. Prior to body composition testing, inform the parents so they will understand the purpose and procedures of this assessment.
2. Instruct students about concepts and procedures for measuring body composition.
3. Maintain records of these measures over time in order to assess the interaction effects of growth, maturation, diet, and physical activity on body composition changes.
4. Measure only standardized sites and follow established procedures.
5. If you feel it is necessary, ask a teacher, nurse, or the child's parent to be present during the body composition testing.
6. Ensure confidentiality by sharing test results with only the child and the parents.
7. Provide personal feedback and group interpretations of the results.
8. Do not use body composition test results for grading purposes.
9. Be sure to make the body composition assessment a positive experience for each child. Do not label, criticize, or ridicule children during any phase of this procedure.

Fat-Free Body Composition of Children

The changes in water, mineral, and protein components of the fat-free body (FFB) due to growth and maturation influence the density of the FFB in children (Boileau et al., 1984; Fomon, Haschke, Ziegler, & Nelson, 1982; Haschke, 1983; Lohman, Slaughter, Boileau, Bunt, & Lussier, 1984). From birth to 22 years of age, the FFB density steadily increases in males from 1.063 to 1.102 g/cc and in females from 1.064 to 1.096 g/cc (Lohman, 1986). The water content of the FFB in children decreases from 79% at 1 year of age to 74% at 20 years of age (Lohman, 1989a). In contrast, the bone mineral content of the FFB in children increases from 3.7% in infants to 6.8% in adulthood (Fomon et al., 1982). Furthermore, when relative body fat is held constant, the overall body density of boys (8 to 10 years of age) is 1.051 g/cc compared to 1.076 g/cc in men (20 to 29 years of age) (Lohman, Slaughter, et al., 1984), reflecting differences in the FFB composition of children and adults.

Thus, the two-component model equations (Brozek et al., 1963; Siri, 1961) underestimate the FFM (1.5 to 2.0 kg) and overestimate the %BF (3% to 4%) in children and youth (Lohman, 1992; Nielsen et al., 1993). Therefore, it is important to select methods and prediction equations based on either multicomponent models or Lohman's (1989a) two-component model conversion formulas that adjust for changes in the FFB density in children (Table 6.1). Nielsen et al. (1993) reported good agreement between a four-component model and Lohman's two-component model estimates of %BF in boys and girls, 8 to 20 years of age.

Table 6.1 Prediction Equations for Children

Method	Ethnicity/gender	Equation	Reference
SKF			
$\Sigma triceps + calf$	Black and White		
	Boys (all ages)	1. $\%BF = 0.735\ (\Sigma SKF) + 1.0$	Slaughter et al. (1988)
	Girls (all ages)	2. $\%BF = 0.610\ (\Sigma SKF) + 5.1$	Slaughter et al. (1988)
$\Sigma triceps + subscapular$ ($\Sigma SKF > 35mm$)	Black and White		
	Boys (all ages)	3. $\%BF = 0.783\ (\Sigma SKF) + 1.6$	Slaughter et al. (1988)
	Girls (all ages)	4. $\%BF = 0.546\ (\Sigma SKF) + 9.7$	Slaughter et al. (1988)
($\Sigma SKF < 35mm$)	Black and White		
	Boys (all ages)	5. $\%BF = 1.21\ (\Sigma SKF) - 0.008\ (\Sigma SKF)^2 + I^*$	Slaughter et al. (1988)
	Girls (all ages)	6. $\%BF = 1.33\ (\Sigma SKF) - 0.013\ (\Sigma SKF)^2 - 2.5$	Slaughter et al. (1988)
BIA	White		
	Boys and girls (6-10 yr)	7. $TBW\ (l)^a = 0.593\ (HT^2/R) + 0.065\ (BW) + 0.04$	Kushner (1992)

(continued)

Table 6.1 (*continued*)

Method	Ethnicity/gender	Equation	Reference
BIA (*continued*)	White		
	Boys and girls (10-19 yr)	8. FFM (kg) = 0.61 (HT²/R) + 0.25 (BW) + 1.31	Houtkooper et al. (1992)
	Boys and girls (8-15 yr)	9. FFM (kg) = 0.62 (HT²/R) + 0.21 (BW) + 0.10 (X$_c$) + 4.2	Lohman (1992)
	Japanese Native		
	Boys (9-14 yr)	10. FFM (kg) = 0.56 (HT²/Z) + 0.20 (BW) + 1.66	Kim et al. (1993)
	Girls (9-15 yr)	11. FFM (kg) = 0.42 (HT²/Z) + 0.60 (BW) – 0.75 (arm C) + 7.72	Watanabe et al. (1993)

ΣSKF = sum of skinfolds (mm), HT = height (cm), BW = body weight (kg), R = resistance (Ω), X$_c$ = reactance (Ω), Z = impedance (Ω), arm C = arm circumference (cm), TBW = total body water (l)

*I = intercept substitutions based on maturation and ethnicity for boys:

Age	Black	White
Prepubescent	–3.2	–1.7
Pubescent	–5.2	–3.4
Postpubescent	–6.8	–5.5

aTo convert TBW to FFM, use the following age-gender hydration constants:

Boys: 5-6 yr FFM (kg) = TBW/0.77   Girls: 5-6 yr FFM (kg) = TBW/0.78
7-8 yr FFM (kg) = TBW/0.768   7-8 yr FFM (kg) = TBW/0.776
9-10 yr FFM (kg) = TBW/0.762   9-10 yr FFM (kg) = TBW/0.77

Skinfold Equations for Children

Age- and race-specific SKF equations for estimating %BF of children were developed by Slaughter et al. (1988) using multicomponent model reference measures. These equations use the sum (Σ) of two skinfolds (triceps + subscapular or triceps + calf SKFs) to predict %BF. The prediction error for these equations ranged from 3.6 %BF to 3.9 %BF. These equations (Table 6.1) may be used to assess the body composition of black and white boys and girls, 8 to 17 years of age. Separate equations were developed for children whose ΣSKF is less than or greater than 35 mm. The intercept of the Σ triceps + subscapular equation for boys varies depending on the maturation stage (prepubescent, pubescent, or postpubescent) of the child.

Recently, Janz et al. (1993) cross-validated the Slaughter SKF equations for girls (Σ triceps + subscapular SKF and Σ triceps + calf SKF equations) and boys (Σ triceps + calf SKF equation). Hydrostatic weighing was used to determine total body density (Db), and Db was converted to %BF using Lohman's (1992) age-gender conversion formulas. For girls, both equations had acceptable prediction errors (SEE = 3.5 %BF to 3.6 %BF). However, the Σ triceps + calf equation slightly overestimated (+1.7 %BF) the average %BF of the girls. For boys, the prediction error for the Σ triceps + calf SKF equation (SEE = 4.6 %BF) was unacceptable and varied with maturation level. Thus, to estimate the %BF of adolescent girls and boys, we suggest using the Σ triceps + subscapular SKF equations (Table 6.1).

Given that the skinfold method requires physical contact with the child, practitioners should be considerate of sensitivity and ethical issues regarding the touching of children by adults. For modest and self-conscious children, particularly young adolescent females, we recommend measuring the triceps and calf SKF sites (Table 6.1) instead of the subscapular site.

The computer software complementing this book selects the appropriate SKF equation based on the age, gender, race, and ΣSKF of the child. In addition, percent body fat charts (Lohman, 1987) can be used to classify levels of body fatness for children (Figure 6.1a-b).

Bioelectrical Impedance Equations for Children

Based on the criteria for selecting prediction equations, the best BIA equation for estimating fat-free mass (FFM) of white boys and girls was developed by Houtkooper et al. (1992), using a three-component model that adjusted body density for total body water (Table 6.1). The equation was cross-validated on samples from three different laboratories, and its prediction error was 2.1 kg. This BIA equation can be used to estimate FFM of boys and girls, ranging in age from 10 to 19 years and in body fatness from 6.5 %BF to 36 %BF. Although Deurenberg, Kusters, and Smit (1990) found that age

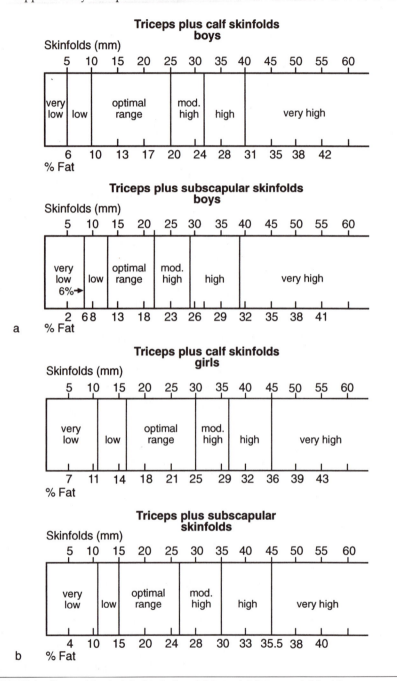

Figure 6.1   Percent body fat charts for children: (a) boys and (b) girls.
Note. From *Measuring Body Fat Using Skinfolds* [videotape] by T.G. Lohman, 1987, Champaign, IL: Human Kinetics. Copyright 1987 by Human Kinetics Publishers. Reprinted with permission.

Table 6.2   Relative Hydration of the Fat-Free Body in Prepubertal Children

| Age (years) | % Water-FFB | |
	Male	Female
5-6	77.0	78.0
7-8	76.8	77.6
9-10	76.2	77.0

Note. Adapted from Lohman (1989a, p. 21).

was significantly related to impedance measures in children, Houtkooper et al. (1992) reported that including age as a predictor did not significantly improve the predictive accuracy of their BIA equation.

To assess the body composition of children younger than 10 years, we recommend using the BIA equations of Lohman (1992) or Kushner, Schoeller, Fjeld, & Danford et al. (1992) (Table 6.1). The Kushner equation estimates the total body water (TBW), instead of FFM, of prepubertal children, ages 6 to 10 years. To develop this equation, the deuterium dilution method was used to obtain reference values for TBW. The prediction error for this equation was 1.41 l. To convert TBW estimates to FFM, Lohman's (1989a) age-gender constants for hydration of the FFB are used (Tables 6.1 and 6.2).

Race-specific BIA equations have been developed and cross-validated for Japanese Native boys (9 to 14 years of age) and girls (9 to 15 years of age) (Kim, Tanaka, Nakadomo, Watanabe, & Matsuura, 1993; Watanabe, Nakadomo, Tanaka, Kim, & Maeda, 1993). These equations have acceptable prediction errors (1.3 to 1.9 kg). Although the equation for Japanese Native girls includes a circumference measure (upper arm), we suggest using it because it is the only equation available for this population subgroup. To date there are no BIA equations that have been developed or cross-validated for American Indian, Asian American, black, or Hispanic children.

Near-Infrared Interactance Equations for Children

At the present time, there is limited research on using the NIR method to estimate body composition of children. The Futrex-5000 NIR analyzer (Model 5000 A) includes equations for children (5 to 12 years) and adolescents (13 to 18 years). Cross-validation of the manufacturer's equations indicated systematic overestimates of the average %BF of children and adolescents by 2.5 %BF to 4.1 %BF. The prediction errors for these equations were large (standard error of estimate or SEE = 4.9 %BF to 5.5 %BF) (Cassady et al.,

1993; Klimis-Tavantis, Oulare, Lehnhard, & Cook, 1992). *Therefore, we do not recommend using these equations to assess body composition of children.*

Anthropometric Equations for Children

Boileau, Wilmore, Lohman, Slaughter, & Riner (1981) developed anthropometric prediction equations using two different samples of boys, ages 8 to 11 years. These equations include combinations of circumferences (arm, wrist, and thigh) and skeletal diameters (wrist and biacromial) to predict body density. The prediction errors for these equations were acceptable (standard error of estimate or SEE = 0.0072 to 0.0075 g/cc); however, they significantly under- or overestimated the average Db in the two samples of children. This difference was attributed to biological variability between the samples and to differences in the methodolgy used to measure residual lung volume. Based on these results, *we do not recommend using these anthropometric equations to assess body composition of children.*

KEY POINTS

■ The SKF and BIA methods can be used to accurately assess the body composition of prepubescent, pubescent, and postpubescent children using the equations of Slaughter et al. (1988), Houtkooper et al. (1992), and Lohman (1992).

■ Race-specific SKF and BIA equations have been developed for black and white children. Also, there is a race-specific BIA equation for Japanese Native children.

■ The NIR and anthropometric methods should not be used to measure body composition of children.

■ Information about body composition should be incorporated in the health and physical-education school curriculum.

■ Health and physical educators need to be concerned about children's privacy and interpret their body composition results in a positive manner.

■ Newly developed prediction equations for the children should be based on multicomponent models to account for interindividual variability in mineral and water components of the FFB.

Chapter 7

Body Composition and the Elderly

Changes in the proportions and densities of the fat-free body (FFB) components due to aging limit the usefulness of the two-component model for estimating the relative body fatness of elderly individuals. With aging, the relative mineral content of the FFB decreases approximately 1% per year between 50 and 70 years of age (Adams, Davis, & Sweetnam, 1970; Smith, Khairi, Norton, & Johnston, 1976). Because of these changes, the density of the FFB in the elderly, particularly elderly women, is less than the assumed value (1.10 g/cc) for the two-component model (Table 1.6). Therefore, prediction equations based on the two-component models of Siri (1961) and Brozek et al. (1963) tend to systematically ovestimate the relative body fat (%BF) in the elderly population by 2% to 4% (Baumgartner et al., 1991). Multicomponent body composition models are recommended for developing prediction equations for the elderly.

In this chapter, body composition methods and prediction equations for elderly men and women are presented (Table 7.1). These equations were se-lected using the criteria outlined in chapter 1. Recommended equations are also summarized in the Quick Reference Guide in Appendix A. To assess the body composition of elderly men and women, the bioelectrical impedance (BIA) method can be used. As an alternative for elderly women, the anthropometric method can be used.

Assessing Body Composition of Elderly

Changes in the FFB composition and the effect of these changes on the density of the FFB in the elderly has not yet been firmly established. Presently,

Table 7.1 Prediction Equations for Elderly

Method	Gender	Equation	Reference
BIA	Women		
	(50-70 yr)	1. FFM (kg) = 0.474 (HT^2/R) + 0.180 (BW) + 7.3	Lohman (1992)
	(22-74 yr)	2. FFM (kg) = 0.00151 (HT^2) – 0.0344 (R) + 0.140 (BW) – 0.158 (age) + 20.387	Gray et al. (1989)
	Men		
	(50-70 yr)	3. FFM (kg) = 0.600 (HT^2/R) + 0.186 (BW) + 0.226 (X_c) – 10.9	Lohman (1992)
	(19-70 yr)	4. FFM (kg) = 0.00139 (HT^2) – 0.0801 (R) + 0.187 (BW) + 39.83	Gray et al. (1989)
	Women		
	(65-94 yr)	5. FFM (kg) = 0.28 (HT^2/R) + 0.27 (BW) + 0.31 (thigh C) – 1.732	Baumgartner et al. (1991)
	Men		
	(65-94 yr)	6. FFM (kg) = 0.28 (HT^2/R) + 0.27 (BW) + 0.31 (thigh C) + 2.768	Baumgartner et al. (1991)
Anthropometry	Women		
	(15-79 yr)	7. Db (g/cc)[a] = 1.168297 – [0.002824 × AB C] + [0.0000122098 × (AB C)²] – [0.000733128 × hip C] + [0.000510477 × HT] – [0.000216161 × age]	Tran & Weltman (1989)

HT = height (cm); BW = body weight (kg); R = resistance (Ω); X_c = reactance (Ω); C = circumference (cm); AB C (cm): average abdominal circumference = $[(AB_1 + AB_2)/2]$, where AB_1 (cm) = abdominal circumference anteriorly midway between the xiphoid process of the sternum and the umbilicus and laterally between the lower end of the rib cage and iliac crests, and AB_2 (cm) = abdominal circumference at the umbilicus level

[a]Use the following formula to convert Db to %BF: %BF = [(5.01/Db) – 4.57] × 100

researchers are trying to determine the amount and direction of changes in the relative proportions and densities of the water, protein, and mineral components of the FFB due to aging. Much of what we know about these factors is speculative because it is based on cross-sectional, rather than longitudinal, studies of the elderly. So far, it appears that the chemical composition of the FFB does not influence the average FFB density in elderly as much as it does in children. However, there is large interindividual variation in the FFB composition of elderly men and women. Therefore, experts recommend using a four-component body composition model to develop prediction equations and to establish reference data for the elderly (Baumgartner et al., 1991; Chumlea & Baumgartner, 1989; Heymsfield et al., 1989; Lohman, 1992).

In addition, the conventional reference method (hydrodensitometry) may need to be modified or replaced by newer methods (e.g., dual-energy x-ray absorptiometry) to obtain accurate reference measures in the elderly (Chumlea & Baumgartner, 1989). Hydrostatic weighing is extremely stressful for some elderly individuals because they may not be able to (a) get in and out of the hydrostatic weighing tank, (b) bend over far enough to be completely submerged because of poor flexibility, and (c) maximally expire all of the air from their lungs for estimation of residual lung volume (RV) and underwater weight. These difficulties could substantially affect the accuracy and measurement error (10 %BF to 15 %BF) of the hydrostatic weighing method (Chumlea & Baumgartner, 1989).

Fat-Free Body Composition of Elderly

Between the ages of 25 and 65 years, there is a substantial decrease in lean body mass (10% to 16%) because of losses in bone mass, skeletal muscle, and total body water with aging (Heymsfield et al., 1989; Kuczmarski, 1989). The change in total body water most likely reflects the loss of intracellular fluid, corresponding to the decline in skeletal muscle mass. Compared to their younger (19 to 34 years of age) counterparts, the mineral, water, and protein components of the FFB in elderly women (> 65 years of age) decline 20%, 12%, and 5%, respectively (Heymsfield et al., 1989). Thus, the relative proportions of the fat-free body components differ for older and younger women: water 71.2% vs. 72.1%, mineral 5.9% vs. 6.5%, and protein 23.0% vs. 21.4%, respectively.

Despite these differences, Heymsfield et al. (1989) reported that the estimated density of the FFB in elderly women is 1.099 g/cc, which is remarkably similar to the value assumed for the two-component model (1.10 g/cc). However, this estimate does not take into account possible changes in bone mineral density with age. Given that bone density decreases at a rate of 1% per year between ages 50 and 70 (Adams et al., 1970; Smith et al., 1976), the actual FFB density of elderly women may be lower than Heymsfield's estimate. Lohman (1992) theoretically estimated the FFB density of elderly women to be 1.0942 g/cc, assuming a 5% decrease in bone mineral density due to aging.

Although the relative body mineral decreases, it is not clear if the relative hydration of the FFB decreases or increases with aging. In contrast to Heymsfield's (1989) data, Baumgartner et al. (1991) found that the relative proportion of water in the fat-free mass (FFM) was higher (74%) in elderly men and women (> 65 years of age), and the estimated fat-free body density was 1.093 and 1.094 g/cc, respectively. Thus, additional research is needed to clarify this point. You should be aware that the formulas reported in chapter 1 (Table 1.6) for converting total body density (Db) to %BF for elderly men and women may be limited. These conversion formulas were calculated using average values, reported in the literature, for FFB density of the elderly derived from four-component models. It is highly likely these formulas will need to be modified once the discrepancy about the hydration of the FFB in the elderly is resolved.

In any event, there is a large degree of variability in the FFB of elderly individuals; therefore, experts advocate using a four-component model to establish reference measures of body composition in this population (Baumgartner et al., 1991; Chumlea & Baumgartner, 1989; Deurenberg, Westrate, & van der Kooy, 1989b). Research indicates that the Siri (1961) (two-component model) equation either under- or overestimated four-component model estimates of %BF in older (49 to 94 years of age) individuals by as much as 10 %BF to 14 %BF (Baumgartner et al., 1991; Williams et al., 1993). On average, the Siri equation systematically overestimated %BF in the elderly by 1 to 3 %BF (Baumgartner et al., 1991; Deurenberg, Westrate, & van der Kooy, 1989b). Unfortunately, there is a limited number of prediction equations based on multicomponent model criterion measures for the elderly population.

Skinfold Equations for Elderly

Durnin and Womersley (1974) published age-specific skinfold (SKF) equations to predict Db of women and men, ranging in age from 16 to 72 years. However, the number of males (N = 24) and females (N = 37) in the older (50+ years) category was limited, and these equations were not cross-validated on separate samples. Also, the prediction errors for older (50+ years) men were large (standard error of estimate or SEE = 0.0090 to 0.0120 g/cc), and only one equation for older women [(log Σ biceps + triceps + subscapular)] had an acceptable prediction error (SEE = 0.0080 g/cc). Broekhoff et al. (1992) reported that the Durnin and Womersley equation significantly overesti-
ated the average FFM of 67- to 78-year-old women by 5.3 kg.

The generalized SKF equations of Jackson et al. (1978, 1980) are based on a quadratic model using the sum of three, four, or seven skinfolds (ΣSKF) and age to predict Db. These equations were developed for men (18 to 61 years of age) and women (18 to 55 years of age), and, therefore, may not be applicable to older individuals exceeding these age ranges. When Jackson et al. applied their equations (Σ3SKFs) to Durnin and Womersley's (1974) samples, there was close agreement (< 1 %BF) between the reference and SKF predicted means in younger women (20 to 40 years of age), but larger differences (3 %BF) in older (40 to 68 years of age) women. Likewise, we found that the Σ3SKF equation significantly underestimated the average %BF of women (40 to 72 years of age) by an average of 3 %BF (unpublished data). Therefore, it appears that these equations should not be used for older women. Similar cross-validation analyses have not been reported for older men.

Williams, Going, Lohman, Hewitt, and Haber (1992) developed SKF equations for white men and women, 60 to 84 years of age. These equations were based on multi-component models that adjusted body density (Db) for bone mineral content and %BF for total body water. The SKF equation for elderly men accurately estimated %BF with an acceptable standard error of estimate (3.3 %BF); for elderly women, the SEE (3.8%) was slightly greater than the recommended value (3.5%). Because these skinfold equations were not cross-validated, we do not recommend using them at this time.

Some experts discourage using the SKF method to assess body composition of elderly clients. With aging, adipose tissue is redistributed, with relatively more subcutaneous and internal fat stored on the trunk than the extremities (Chumlea & Baumgartner, 1989). Age-related decreases in the elasticity and hydration of the skin, as well as shrinkage in the size of fat cells, may increase the compressibility of subcutaneous adipose and connective tissues (Kuczmarski, 1989). Experts, therefore, recommend using alternative methods, such as circumference measures or BIA, to estimate body composition in the elderly.

Bioelectrical Impedance Equations for Elderly

There are relatively few age-specific bioelectrical impedance (BIA) equations to predict body composition in the elderly (Baumgartner et al., 1991; Deurenberg et al., 1990; Lohman, 1992). Deurenberg, van der Kooy, Evers, & Hulshof (1990) developed a BIA equation for 60- to 83-year-old men and women but failed to cross-validate it. Although Broekhoff et al. (1992) found that this equation accurately estimated the average fat-free mass (FFM) of 67- to 78-year-old women (standard error of estimate or SEE = 2.2 kg), others have reported that this equation systematically underestimates FFM (by 5.0 kg) and overestimates fat mass (by 10 kg) in elderly women (Jenkins et al., 1994; Svendsen, Haarbo, Heitmann, Gotfredsen, & Christiansen, 1991).

Some age-specific BIA equations are based on multicomponent models, correcting for interindividual variability in either bone mineral content and/or total body water. Lohman's (1992) equations (Table 7.1) for the elderly (50 to 70 years of age) estimate FFM, adjusted for bone mineral, with an acceptable degree of accuracy (SEE = 3.0 kg in men and 2.8 kg in women). Cross-validation of the elderly equation on another sample of older women (50 to 70 years of age) yielded small differences in FFM (< 0.8 kg) and good predictive accuracy (SEE = 2.1 to 2.4 kg) (Jenkins et al., 1994; Wilson et al., 1992). We recommend using Lohman's (50 to 70 years) equation to assess body composition of elderly women; however, further study is needed to confirm the predictive accuracy of the equation for elderly men (50 to 70 years).

Baumgartner's (1991) age-specific BIA equation (Table 7.1) may be applicable for assessing the body composition of very elderly women and men (65 to 94 years of age). This equation was developed using a four-component model, correcting Db for total body water and total body mineral, and a jackknife regression procedure. Briefly, this procedure randomly selects subsamples from the total sample and generates prediction equations for each subsample. Data from these equations are averaged to provide a more stable prediction equation. Although the jackknife procedure is not a substitute for cross-validation analysis, the original validation statistics (SEE = 2.5 kg) are promising; however, this equation still needs to be cross-validated on additional samples of elderly women and men before we can recommend using it.

There are gender-specific, generalized BIA equations (Table 7.1), based on two-component model estimates of FFM, that may be applicable to the elderly (Gray et al., 1989). Although these equations were not cross-validated in Gray's study, we found that the generalized equation for women accurately predicted the FFM of 20- to 72-year-old women (SEE = 2.4 kg), with no significant difference between criterion and predicted FFM (Jenkins et al., 1994). When we tested this equation on only those women between 50 and 72 years of age, similar results were noted (SEE = 2.4 kg), and the difference between reference and predicted FFM was < 1 kg.

In summary, *we recommend using either Lohman's age-specific (50 to 70 years) equation or Gray's generalized equation to estimate FFM of elderly women.* However, because these equations have not been adequately cross-validated for men, we cannot say for certain they will accurately estimate the FFM of your elderly, male clients.

Near-Infrared Interactance Equations for Elderly

As discussed in chapter 4, much more research needs to be done before ⁀ near-infrared interactance (NIR) method can be applied to population subgroups such as elderly women and men. We advise against using the Futrex-5000 manufacturer's NIR equation because of its poor predictive accuracy. Also, the NIR equation (Heyward, Jenkins, et al., 1992), developed and cross-validated for women varying in age (20 to 72 years), needs to be tested on other samples before we can recommend using it for elderly women. *Therefore, we suggest you use alternative field methods, like BIA and anthropometric equations, to assess body composition of your elderly clients.*

Anthropometric Equations for Elderly

Generalized anthropometric equations (Table 7.1) have been developed for estimating Db from circumference measurements in women (15 to 79 years) and men (21 to 78 years) (Tran & Weltman, 1988, 1989). Cross-validation of these equations indicated that the predictive accuracy for the female equation (standard error of estimate or SEE = 0.0082 g/cc) was good, but the SEE for the male equation (0.0107 g/cc) was poor. Thus, we do not recommend using this equation to estimate the Db of elderly men. In the anthropometric equation for women, the average of two abdominal circumferences, hip circumference, height, and age are used to predict Db. The two circumferences are measured (a) midway between the xiphoid process of the sternum and the umbilicus, and (b) at the level of the umbilicus. To obtain %BF estimates from Db for elderly women, use the appropriate age-gender conversion formula (Table 7.1).

KEY POINTS

- Lohman's (1992) age-specific BIA equations or Gray's (1989) generalized equation may be used to assess the body composition of elderly women and men.
- Tran and Weltman's (1989) generalized anthropometric equation may be used to assess the body composition of elderly women; the equation for men needs further cross-validation.
- SKF and NIR methods should not be used to assess body composition in the elderly.
- Additional research is needed to cross-validate existing BIA equations, especially for elderly men. The equations of Lohman (1992), Gray et al. (1989), and Baumgartner et al. (1991) are good candidates for cross-validation.

Chapter 8

Body Composition and Ethnicity

There are strong links between ethnicity, obesity, and disease. The prevalence of overweight and obesity in the United States varies from 24% to 75%, depending on race (U.S. Department of Health and Human Services, 1990). Certain ethnic groups have a relatively higher risk for obesity, predisposing them to cardiovascular disease, hypertension, noninsulin-dependent diabetes mellitis (NIDDM), certain cancers, and osteoarthritis. For this reason, population subgroups, particularly black women, Hispanic women, and American Indian women and men, have been targeted for weight loss in the Healthy People 2000 National Health Promotion and Disease Prevention Objectives (U.S. Department of Health and Human Services, 1990). As such, there is a need for practical methods and equations that can be used to accurately assess the degree of adiposity of individuals from different ethnic origins.

Crude indexes of total body fatness, such as body mass index (BMI) and abdominal obesity (waist-to-hip ratio or WHR), fail to identify at-risk individuals and do not always accurately predict all-cause mortality in certain ethnic groups (Stevens et al., 1992). For example, we found that only 25% of American Indian women in our sample were identified as obese using body mass index (BMI > 27.8). In contrast, 78% were classified as obese (≥ 32 %BF) using hydrodensitometry and a three-component body composition model to estimate the body fat of these women. This illustrates the importance of using more precise and accurate methods for assessing body composition and identifying individuals at-risk due to obesity.

Body Composition and Health Risks of American Indians

Noninsulin-dependent diabetes mellitus (NIDDM) or Type II diabetes is a major cause of death and morbidity in the American Indian population (Welty, 1991). The age-adjusted death rate from diabetes is 2.4 times greater than that of all other ethnic groups (U.S. Department of Health and Human Services, 1990). Likewise, the risk of developing NIDDM is 10.8 times greater for American Indians compared with the white population (Carter Center of Emory University, 1985). The prevalence of diabetes is especially high for American Indians living in the southwestern region of the United States. For example, the Pima Indians in Arizona have the highest reported prevalence of NIDDM in the world (Knowler, Pettitt, Savage, & Bennett, 1981).

There is a strong association between obesity and NIDDM. Over the past 30 years, the prevalence of obesity in American Indians has escalated. Based on BMI data obtained from the 1987 National Medical Expenditure Survey, Broussard et al. (1991) estimated that approximately 14% of American Indian men and 17% of American Indian women are obese. In addition, 34% of the men and 40% of the women in this group are overweight. These values exceeded those reported for all other ethnic groups in the United States. However, crude indexes of obesity, like body mass index (BMI), fail to identify many at-risk individuals. Thus, the prevalence of obesity in the American Indian population may be much higher than that reported by Broussard et al. (1991).

Body Composition and Health Risks of Blacks

Although the prevalence of obesity in black men is similar to that of white men, this is not the case for black women. Throughout the life span, the prevalence of obesity in black women is twice that of white women. Based on a large epidemiological survey, 30% of younger (18-30 years) and 77% of older (45-65 years) black women were obese compared to 14% and 46%, respectively, for their white counterparts (Folsom et al., 1991). In a 10-year longitudinal study of obesity, black women reportedly were 60% more likely to become obese than white women (Williamson, Kahn, & Byers, 1991).

In addition, Folsom et al. (1991) reported that obesity is related to elevated cardiovascular risk factors in the black population. In 18- to 30-year-old blacks, obesity was associated with a 1.5-fold increase in hypercholesterolemia, a twofold increase in hypertension, and a fourfold increase in diabetes.

Body Composition and Health Risks of Hispanics

The prevalence of obesity and overweight in the U.S. Hispanic population is similar to that of American Indians. Based on body mass index (BMI) and the sum of two skinfolds, Pawson, Martorell, and Mendoza (1991) reported that the prevalence of overweight for Hispanic men and women was, respectively, 36% and 42% for Mexican Americans in the Southwest, 31% and 41% for Puerto Ricans in the New York City area, and 34% and 38% for Cubans in Florida.

High levels of obesity in the Hispanic population are associated with elevated risk for cardiovascular and metabolic diseases in this ethnic group (Gaskill, Allen, Garza, Gonzales, & Waldrop, 1981; Haffner, Stern, Mitchell, Hazuda, & Patterson, 1990). Samet, Coultas, Howard, Skipper, and Hanis (1988) suggested that Mexican Americans and American Indians in the Southwest may share the same genetic component responsible for obesity and related metabolic disorders. Because the Hispanic population is the fastest growing minority group in the United States, it is reasonable to speculate that the prevalence of obesity-linked diseases will also increase, placing a relatively greater burden on the public health care system (Pawson et al., 1991).

Body Composition and Health Risks of Asians

The prevalence of obesity in Japanese American (13%) and Japanese Native (3%) men is low; however, the relatively higher prevalence in Japanese Americans reflects the impact of Westernization on lifestyle, diet, and obesity for Japanese in the United States. For example, Japanese men in Hawaii and California have a higher body mass index (BMI) and skinfold thicknesses than Japanese Natives (Curb & Marcus, 1991). Recently, Wang, Thornton, Burastero, Heymsfield, and Pierson (1995) reported an average %BF of 21% for an Asian American sample of men who were predominantly Chinese (93% of sample).

Although Japanese men are relatively lean, this does not appear to be the case for women. The average %BF of Japanese American women reportedly was 33%, 35%, and 33%, respectively, for younger (20 to 29 years), middle-aged (40 to 59 years), and older (70 to 79 years) women. Similar data were noted for younger (32 %BF), middle-aged (36 %BF), and older (31 %BF) women in Japan (Tsunenari et al., 1993) and Asian women (32 %BF), ages 18 to 94 years, in the United States (Wang et al., 1994, 1995).

Although the Asian populations in the United States and Japan have a relatively lower risk for cardiovascular and metabolic diseases, osteoporosis is a serious disease afflicting some Asian populations, especially women. The average bone mineral content and bone density of Japanese, Chinese, and Korean women is lower than overall values reported for women in the United States and Europe (Hagiwara et al., 1989; Sugimoto et al., 1992; Tsai, Huang, Chieng, & Cheng, 1991). Although the average total body bone mineral density of Japanese American and Japanese Native women did not differ, Japanese American women (20 to 60 years) had a lower bone mineral density (1.101 g/cm^2) compared to American Indian women (1.175 g/cm^2) of the same age (Kin et al., 1992; McHugh et al., 1993). These findings explain, in part, the relatively greater risk for developing osteoporosis in some Asian populations.

Body Composition and Health Risks of Whites

Although obesity is a relatively greater problem in minority populations, approximately one out of every four white adults in the United States is overweight (Kuczmarski, 1992). Thus, overweight and obesity is also a serious health problem in the white population. The prevalence of hypertension, hyperlipidemia, and Type II diabetes are, respectively, 2.9, 2.1 and 2.9 times greater in overweight than normal-weight individuals (National Institutes of Health, 1985). Cardiovascular disease remains the leading cause of death, accounting for almost one half of all deaths in the United States (American Heart Association, 1994).

Presently, research is focused on quantifying the fat-free body (FFB) composition of certain ethnic populations. In the past, research dealing with ethnic differences in FFB composition was hampered by the lack of suitable technologies to quantify these relationships. However, recent technological advances, such as dual-energy x-ray absorptiometry, have overcome this problem by providing reasonably accurate estimates of bone mineral, soft tissue, and lean tissue mass. Because this area of investigation is relatively new, there is a limited number of race-specific prediction equations based on multicomponent body composition models.

In this chapter, body composition methods suitable for American Indians, blacks, Hispanics, Japanese Natives, and white population subgroups are summarized in Table 8.1. Recommended equations for each ethnic group are also presented in Tables 8.2 through 8.6 and in the Quick Reference Guide in Appendix A. These ethnic-specific equations were chosen using the selection criteria outlined in chapter 1. For some ethnic groups, equations are based on multicomponent models that take into account variability in the water and mineral content of the FFB. In addition, we recommend using race-specific conversion formulas (Table 1.6) to convert Db to %BF for individuals from specific ethnic groups.

Assessing Body Composition of American Indians

Because of the high prevalence of NIDDM and obesity in the American Indian population, this population has been targeted for weight loss. In this

Table 8.1   Summary of Body Composition Methods Applicable to Ethnic Groups

Population		SKF	BIA	NIR	Anthropometry
American Indian	Male		✔		
	Female	✔	✔	✔	
Black	Male	✔			
	Female	✔			
Hispanic	Male		✔		
	Female	✔	✔	✔	
Japanese Native	Male	✔	✔		
	Female	✔	✔		
White	Male	✔	✔		✔
	Female	✔	✔	✔	✔

section, information about the fat-free body composition of American Indians is presented. Also, methods and equations that can be used to assess the body composition of American Indian men and women are summarized in Tables 8.1 and 8.2.

Fat-Free Body Composition of American Indians

Although the components (water, mineral, and protein) of the FFB have not been investigated for American Indian men and children, McHugh et al. (1993) found that the average bone mineral density (1.18 g/cm^2) and bone mineral content (2596 g) of American Indian women were significantly greater than age-matched reference data. The average relative total body mineral of American Indian women was 8.1% of the fat-free mass (FFM), compared to 6.8% FFM assumed for the reference body. In fact, American Indian women have one of the highest relative, total body mineral values reported in the literature to date (Stolarczyk et al., 1994). Based on this value, the density of the FFB for American Indian women was estimated to be 1.108 g/cc (Table 1.6). Therefore, use of two-component model equations will significantly underestimate the %BF of American Indian women.

Skinfold Equations for American Indians

Unfortunately, existing SKF prediction equations have not been cross-validated on populations of American Indian men. Therefore, we cannot recommend using the SKF method for estimating the body composition of men at this time. Hicks, Heyward, Flores, et al. (1993) cross-validated the Jackson

Table 8.2 Prediction Equations for American Indians

Method	Gender	Equation	Reference
SKF (triceps + midaxillary + suprailiac)	Women (18-60 yr)	1. Db (g/cc)^a = 1.061983 − 0.000385 (ΣSKF) − 0.000204 (age)	Hicks, Heyward, Flores, et al. (1993)
BIA	Women (18-60 yr)	2. FFM (kg) = 0.1555 (BW) + 0.001254 (HT^2) − 0.04904 (R) + 0.1417 (X_c) − 0.0833 (age) + 20.05	Stolarczyk et al. (1994)
	Men (18-29 yr)	3. FFM (kg) = 0.485 (HT^2/R) + 0.338 (BW) + 5.32	Lohman (1992)
	(30-49 yr)	4. FFM (kg) = 0.549 (HT^2/R) + 0.163 (BW) + 0.092 (X_c) + 4.51	Lohman (1992)
	(50-70 yr)	5. FFM (kg) = 0.60 (HT^2/R) + 0.186 (BW) + 0.226 (X_c) − 10.9	Lohman (1992)
NIR (pectoral + biceps)	Women (18-60 yr)	6. Db (g/cc)^a = 1.070761 − 0.000987 (hip C) − 0.036986 ($\Sigma\Delta OD_2$) + 0.000417 (HT) + 0.000087 (FIT index) − 0.000189 (age)	Hicks, Heyward, Flores, et al. (1993)

ΣSKF = sum of skinfold (mm), BW = body weight (kg), HT = height (cm), R = resistance (Ω), X_c = reactance (Ω), hip C = hip circumference (cm), $\Sigma\Delta OD_2$ = [(OD$_2$ standard − OD$_2$ pectoral) + (OD$_2$ standard − OD$_2$ biceps)], FIT index = physical activity level (see Figure 8.1, page 112)

[a] Use the following formula to convert Db to %BF: %BF = [(4.81/Db) − 4.34] × 100

FIT Index

Ask your client the following questions and circle the corresponding number:
- Frequency (F)—How many days per week do you exercise?
- Intensity (I)—What type of physical activities do you participate in?
- Time (T)—How many minutes is your exercise workout?

Frequency	5	6 or 7 times per week
	4	3 to 5 times per week
	3	1 or 2 times per week
	2	A few times per month
	1	Less than once per month
Intensity	5	High intensity activities that result in sustained heavy breathing and perspiration (e.g., high impact aerobics, running, speed swimming, distance cycling).
	4	Moderately high aerobic activities and intermittent sports activities that result in sustained heavy breathing and perspiration (e.g., step aerobics, stairstepping, speed walking, tennis, racquetball, squash).
	3	Moderate aerobic activities (e.g., normal bike riding, jogging, low impact aerobics).
	2	Low to moderate aerobic and sports activities (e.g., recreational volleyball, moderate speed walking).
	1	Light aerobic activities (e.g., normal walking, golfing).
Time	4	Over 30 minutes
	3	20-30 minutes
	2	10-20 minutes
	1	Under 10 minutes

Calculate FIT index by multiplying F × I × T (scores can range from 1 to 100)

Figure 8.1 FIT index for assessing physical activity level.
Note. From "The Effects of Exercise and Fitness on Serum Lipids in College Women" (p. 46), by D. Kasari, 1976, unpublished master's thesis, University of Montana. Adapted with permission.

---

et al. (1980) sum of seven skinfolds (Σ7SKF) and (Σ3SKF) equations in a group of 150 American Indian women from New Mexico and found strong, positive relationships ($r = 0.82$ to 0.83) between measured and predicted Db for both equations. However, there was a significant underestimation of the average measured Db. Additionally, the SEEs for the Σ7SKF (0.0081 g/cc) and Σ3SKF (0.0085 g/cc) equations slightly exceeded the recommended upper limit (0.0080 g/cc). These equations may have failed to accurately predict

Db due to differences in subcutaneous fat distribution between American Indian and white women. Hicks (1992) reported that in comparison to white women, American Indian women tend to deposit more fat on the trunk than on the extremities.

Therefore, a SKF equation for American Indian women, based on a three-component model that adjusted Db for total body mineral, was developed. This equation was cross-validated on a sample of 50 American Indian women. The prediction error for this equation was excellent (SEE = 0.0068 g/cc), and there was no significant difference between the measured and SKF-predicted Db means. Therefore, *we recommend using the Hicks, Heyward, Flores et al. (1993) equation for estimating the Db of American Indian women, 18 to 60 years of age* (Table 8.2). To convert Db into %BF, we suggest using the race-specific conversion formula for American Indian women (Table 8.2).

Bioelectrical Impedance Equations for American Indians

BIA is one clinical method that is widely used on reservations and pueblos for assessing body composition of American Indians. Because some American Indians are severely obese, it may not be possible to accurately measure their skinfold thicknesses. Therefore, the BIA method may be a more suitable field method for body composition assessment in this population.

Rising et al. (1991) developed a race-specific BIA prediction equation for Pima Indians (men and women) who varied greatly in body fatness (11 %BF to 52 %BF). When cross-validated, this equation was found to be superior to Lukaski's (1986) gender-specific equations in estimating reference FFM (SEE = 3.2 kg vs. 6.9 kg, respectively). However, the Rising race-specific equation was developed using the Keys and Brozek (1953) two-component model formula to estimate reference FFM. The Keys and Brozek equation was theoretically derived using hypothetical values for relative body fatness (14 %BF for body density = 1.063 g/cc) of a "reference man." Later, Brozek et al. (1963) revised this equation based on empirical data for a reference body (15.3 %BF for Db = 1.064 g/cc). Thus, the Keys and Brozek equation systematically underestimates fat content at any given Db compared to the revised Brozek equation.

We examined the predictive accuracy of the Rising equation in 71 American Indians (40 women, 31 men) in New Mexico. Although the prediction error (SEE = 3.1 kg) was good and there was no significant difference between predicted and reference FFM, the average FFM estimated by this equation was significantly greater than the average FFM estimated by the Brozek et al. (1963), Siri (1961), and Lohman (1992) age-gender conversion formulas (Hicks, Wilson, & Heyward, 1992). Our data indicated that the Rising equation underestimates the average %BF of American Indian men by approximately 2 %BF to 3 %BF.

Subsequently, we assessed the predictive accuracy of other BIA equations (Gray et al., 1989; Lohman, 1992; Segal et al., 1988; Van Loan & Mayclin, 1987) for estimating FFM of American Indian men (Heyward, Wilson, & Stolarczyk, 1994). The Lohman age-specific equations and the generalized equation of Van Loan accurately estimated average FFM with acceptable prediction errors (E = 2.5 to 3.1 kg). All of the other BIA equations significantly underestimated the FFM of American Indian men. Because the prediction error for the Van Loan equation was slightly larger (0.6 kg) than that of the Lohman equations, *we recommend using the Lohman equations* (Table 8.2). However, given that the total body bone mineral of American Indian women is substantially higher than that of other ethnic groups, there is reason to believe that American Indian men may also have an increased bone mineral content. Although we have no data to support this hypothesis, the practitioner should be advised that the Lohman age-specific equations may underestimate the relative body fat of American Indian men because these equations were derived using two-component model reference measures.

In another study involving 151 American Indian women (Stolarczyk et al., 1994), we cross-validated the Rising equation against a three-component model that adjusted Db for total body mineral. The Rising equation overestimated average FFM in this sample by almost 4 kg. Additionally, this equation failed to correctly identify 30% of the women in our sample who were obese (≥ 32 %BF).

Therefore, we generated a new race-specific BIA equation to estimate FFM of American Indian women (18 to 60 years) with a wide range of body fatness (14 %BF to 57 %BF). Cross-validation of this equation on a subsample from this population indicated good predictive accuracy (SEE = 2.6 kg), and there was no significant difference between three-component model reference values and BIA-predicted FFM. Although this equation needs to be cross-validated on additional samples of American Indian women, *we recommend using the Stolarcyzk et al. (1994) equation to estimate FFM of American Indian women, ages 18 to 60 years* (Table 8.2).

Near-Infrared Interactance Equations for American Indians

As with the SKF method, the NIR method cannot be used to assess body composition of American Indian men. We cross-validated the Futrex-5000 NIR manufacturer's equation on a small sample of American Indian men from the Southwest. This equation had a large, systematic prediction error (SEE = 8.3 %BF) and significantly underestimated average %BF of this sample by 2.4 %BF (unpublished observations).

In addition, Hicks, Heyward, Flores, et al. (1993) cross-validated a multisite NIR equation (Heyward, Jenkins, et al., 1992) and the Futrex-5000 manufacturer's NIR equation for a sample of American Indian women (18 to 60 years of age). Prediction errors for both the Heyward equation and the Futrex-5000 equation exceeded 0.0080 g/cc or 3.5 %BF. In addition, the multisite equation significantly overestimated the average body density, and the Futrex-5000 equation significantly underestimated %BF. Therefore, a new NIR equation, based on a multicomponent model, was developed and cross-validated (Table 8.2). This new equation yielded an acceptable prediction error (SEE = 0.0076 g/cc) and small, but significant, differences between NIR-predicted and measured Db.

Although we prefer using the race-specific SKF and BIA equations, rather than this NIR equation to assess body composition of American Indian women, the NIR method may be used if it is the only available method in your clinical setting. However, *we do not recommend using the Futrex-5000 manufacturer's equation or Heyward's multisite NIR equation for this population.*

Anthropometric Equations for American Indians

There are no anthropometric equations that have been developed or cross-validated for American Indians. Therefore, alternative methods, like BIA or SKF, should be used.

Assessing Body Composition of Blacks

Because excess adiposity is detrimental to cardiovascular health of the black population, it is important to be able to assess levels of body fatness for accurate screening of at-risk individuals. In this section, body composition methods and equations applicable to the black population are presented in Table 8.3.

Fat-Free Body Composition of Blacks

Research demonstrates that the FFB composition of blacks differs from that of whites. Black men and women have relatively greater skeletal muscle mass, bone mineral mass, and bone density than whites (Cohn et al., 1977; Nelson, Feingold, Bolin, & Parfitt, 1991; Ortiz et al., 1992; Schutte et al., 1984). Thus, the estimated density of the FFB is 1.113 g/cc for black men and 1.106 g/cc for black women.

Although the relative hydration of the FFB is similar for blacks and whites (~74% for women and ~73% for men), the relative mineral content in the FFB of younger (7.8%) and middle-aged (7.5%) black women is somewhat higher than that of their white counterparts (7.3% and 6.7%, respectively, for younger and middle-aged white women) (Deck-Cote & Adams, 1993; Ortiz et al., 1992). Also, the average bone mineral density of black women

Table 8.3 . Prediction Equations for Blacks

Method	Gender	Equation	Reference
SKF (*chest + abdomen + thigh + triceps + subscapular + suprailiac + midaxillary*)	Women (18-55 yr)	1. Db $(g/cc)^a$ = 1.0970 − 0.00046971 $(\Sigma 7SKF)$ + 0.00000056 $(\Sigma 7SKF)^2$ − 0.00012828 (age)	Jackson et al. (1980)
	Men (18-61 yr)	2. Db $(g/cc)^a$ = 1.1120 − 0.00043499 $(\Sigma 7SKF)$ + 0.00000055 $(\Sigma 7SKF)^2$ − 0.00028826 (age)	Jackson & Pollock (1978)

$\Sigma 7SKF$ = sum of seven skinfolds (mm)

[a] Use the following formulas to convert Db to %BF: Men %BF = [(4.37/Db) − 3.93] × 100, Women %BF = [(4.85/Db) − 4.39] × 100

(1.18 to 1.25 g/cm^2) is significantly greater than that of white women (1.09 to 1.16 g/cm^2) (Deck-Cote & Adams, 1993; Ortiz et al., 1992).

Compared to multicomponent estimates of body fat, the Siri two-component model equation systematically underestimates the average relative body fat of black women and men by 2 %BF to 3 %BF (Ortiz et al., 1992; Schutte et al., 1984). In contrast, Deck-Cote & Adams (1993) reported very close agreement between multicomponent and two-component model estimates of %BF in young black women, suggesting that the FFB density of these women is close to 1.10 g/cc. This points to the importance of using prediction equations based on multicomponent models to account for variability in bone mineral content and bone density between samples and individuals from the same racial group.

Skinfold Equations for Blacks

Some researchers have reported that the relationship between SKF and body density differs for black and white men (Schutte et al., 1984; Vickery, Cureton, & Collins, 1988). Based on this observation, Vickery developed a race-specific SKF equation for black males, 18 to 32 years of age. The standard error of estimate for this equation was good (0.0070 g/cc); however, it was not cross-validated on a separate sample from this population. Although Vickery measured the same seven skinfolds used in the generalized SKF equation of Jackson and Pollock (1978), they did not test the predictive accuracy of this equation for their sample. When we substituted the average sum of seven skinfolds (Σ7SKF) and age of the black men in Vickery's study into Jackson and Pollock's equation, the predicted body density (1.0744 g/cc) was almost identical to the measured Db (1.075 g/cc). However, we could not evaluate the prediction error for this equation without the individual subject data. Until Vickery's race-specific equation is cross-validated on additional samples of black men, we cannot recommend its use.

Schutte et al. (1984) reported that the average Db, estimated from six different age-specific SKF equations for men, was significantly underestimated in black men, 18 to 32 years of age. However, Hortobagyi, Israel, Houmard, McCammon, et al. (1992) observed no differences in %BF estimated from Jackson and Pollock's Σ7SKF equation for a multi-ethnic sample (black and white) in which 30% of the subjects were young, black men. Also, they found that this equation accurately predicted (SEE = 2.2 %BF) average body fatness of black football players (Hortobagyi, Israel, Houmard, O'Brien et al., 1992). In these two studies, reference %BF was calculated from Db using the Schutte et al. (1984) race-specific conversion formula (Table 1.6).

Because the relationship between SKFs and %BF is similar for black and white women (Slaughter et al., 1988), the average %BF of black women, estimated from the Siri two-component model equation, was accurately predicted (SEE = 3.5 %BF) using the Jackson, Pollock, and Ward (1980) generalized (Σ7SKF) equation (Sparling, Millard-Stafford, Rosskopf, Di-Carlo, & Hinson, 1993). This finding also lends support to Deck-Cote and Adams' (1993) observation that the FFB density of black women is similar to that of the reference body (1.10 g/cc).

In contrast, Zillikens and Conway (1990) reported that the Σ7SKF equation systematically underestimated the average %BF of black women, 19 to 44 years of age, by 3 %BF; however, in this study, total body water, measured by deuterium dilution, was used to estimate fat-free mass (FFM = TBW/0.73) instead of hydrodensitometry. This could explain the disparity between studies.

Based on these findings, *we recommend using the Σ7SKF equations (Jackson & Pollock, 1978; Jackson et al., 1980) to predict Db for your black clients.* However, the race-specific conversion formulas (Table 8.3) should be used to estimate %BF from Db in this population, particularly black men.

Bioelectrical Impedance Equations for Blacks

Recent research indicates that age-specific and generalized BIA equations significantly underestimate the average fat-free mass in black women and men by as much as 3 to 14 kg (Hortobagyi, Israel, Houmard, O'Brien, et al. 1992; Sparling et al., 1993; Zillikens and Conway, 1990). Sparling et al. (1993) tested the predictive accuracy of the Lukaski, Bolonchuk, Hall, and Siders (1986) gender-specific BIA equation that was developed using a sample of white women, 19 to 43 years of age. This equation systematically underestimated FFM of black women by 4 kg. Also, the prediction error for this equation (SEE = 4.0 kg) was unacceptable.

Similarly, Hortobagyi, Israel, Houmard, O'Brien, et al. (1992) examined the predictive accuracy of several BIA equations (Deurenberg, Westrate, & van der Kooy, 1989a; Gray et al., 1989; Heitmann, 1990; Lukaski et al., 1985; Segal et al., 1988) developed for white men. With the exception of Deurenberg's equation, these equations had acceptable prediction errors ($\leq$ 3.5 kg); however, each equation systematically underestimated the average FFM of black, collegiate football players.

Recently, we cross-validated previously published BIA equations (Gray et al., 1989; Lohman, 1992; Rising et al., 1991; Segal et al., 1988; Van Loan & Mayclin, 1987) for a sample of black men (Heyward, Wilson, & Stolarczyk, 1994). Each of these equations systematically underestimated average FFM by 1.5 to 5.1 kg, and the prediction errors were unacceptable (E = 3.1 to 6.0 kg). These findings suggest that race-specific BIA equations need to be developed for black men and women.

There are several reasons why these BIA equations underestimate FFM in blacks:

1. Differences in body proportions may affect the relationship between the resistance index [height squared (HT^2)/resistance (R)] and FFM.

Blacks, on the average, tend to have relatively shorter trunks and longer limbs than whites (Malina, 1973). Because total body resistance is largely determined by segmental resistances in the extremities, the total body resistance will be greater in blacks compared to whites, resulting in an underestimate of FFM.

2. The skeletal muscle mass and bone mass in the limbs is relatively greater in blacks than whites. Therefore, it is incorrect to assume that the specific resistivity of the body is the same for blacks and whites. Recently, Stokes, Sinning, Morgan, and Ellison (1993) reported that the specific resistivity of the lower limbs is significantly greater in black women compared to white women, reflecting differences in the tissue composition in the lower extremity.

3. The amount of bone comprising the FFM is relatively greater in blacks than whites, thereby influencing the cross-sectional area of the FFM and the body's geometry.

4. Blacks have a relatively greater amount of FFM per unit of height (Vickery et al., 1988), suggesting that the relationship between HT^2/R and FFM will differ for black and white populations.

These findings explain, in part, why BIA equations, developed primarily using white samples, significantly underestimate the FFM in blacks. Therefore, until race-specific BIA equations are developed for black men and women, *we cannot recommend using the BIA method to estimate body composition of your black clients.*

Near-Infrared Interactance Equations for Blacks

Presently, the NIR method and the Futrex-5000 manufacturer's equation should not be used to assess body composition in the black population. We cross-validated the manufacturer's equation on a sample of black men. The average body fat was significantly underestimated by 3.7 %BF, and the prediction error (SEE = 4.0 %BF) was large (unpublished observations).

For a mixed sample of black and white men, Hortobagyi, Israel, Houmard, McCammon, et al. (1992) reported slightly better results using the combination of body weight, height, physical activity, and the average optical density (OD) values from eight sites to predict %BF (SEE = 3.6 %BF). This NIR model underestimated the average body fat of their sample by less than 1 %BF. However, the equation was not reported or cross-validated. Also, in two samples of black, collegiate football players, the manufacturer's NIR equation underestimated body fat by 2.1 %BF to 7.2 %BF, on the average (SEE = 3.7 %BF to 3.9 %BF) (Hortobagyi, Israel, Houmard, O'Brien, et al., 1992; Houmard et al., 1991).

In short, *we do not recommend using the NIR method to estimate body composition of your black clients.* Additional research is needed to develop race-specific

NIR equations for this population. It is highly probable the relationship between biceps OD and %BF differs for blacks and whites because blacks have relatively larger arm circumferences (Stevens et al., 1992), lesser subcutaneous fat at the biceps site (Mueller, Shoup, & Malina, 1982; Zillikens & Conway, 1990), and darker skintones (Wilson & Heyward, 1993a) than whites.

Anthropometric Equations for Blacks

Our search of the literature did not uncover any anthropometric prediction equations developed specifically for blacks or any generalized anthropometric equations that are applicable to this group. However, in black and white children, different combinations of anthropometric measures (skinfolds, circumferences, and skeletal diameters) were associated with total body density, depending on race and gender (Harsha, Frerichs, & Berenson, 1978). This finding most likely reflects ethnic differences in skeletal size and muscle mass and suggests that *race-specific anthropometric equations need to be developed before this method can be used to estimate body composition in the black population.*

Assessing Body Composition of Hispanics

Although there is a great need for information concerning appropriate methods for body fat assessment in Hispanics, there are few published research studies on this topic. Data from one study suggest that race-specific equations should be developed in order to accurately estimate minimal wrestling weight of Hispanic and non-Hispanic high school wrestlers (Roby, Kempema, Lohman, Williams, & Tipton, 1991). In the future, this line of investigation needs to be pursued and expanded for the entire Hispanic population. In this section, the FFB composition of Hispanic women is described, as well as body composition methods and equations applicable to the Hispanic population (Table 8.4).

Fat-Free Body Composition of Hispanics

Despite the fact that the Hispanic population is the second largest minority group in the United States (Pawson et al., 1991), there has been no research reported on the fat-free body composition or race-specific prediction equations for this population. In most cases, we were unable to ascertain whether or not Hispanics were included in the original samples that were used to develop the body composition equations presented in this chapter. Although

Table 8.4 Prediction Equations for Hispanics

Method	Gender	Equation	Reference
SKF (chest + abdomen + thigh + triceps + subscapular + suprailiac + midaxillary)	Women (20-40 yr)	1. Db $(g/cc)^a$ = 1.0970 − 0.00046971 (Σ7SKF) + 0.00000056 $(\Sigma 7SKF)^2$ − 0.00012828 (age)	Jackson et al. (1980)
BIA	Women (20-40 yr)	2. FFM (kg) = 0.00151 (HT^2) − 0.0344 (R) + 0.140 (BW) − 0.158 (age) + 20.387	Gray et al. (1989)
	Men (19-59 yr)	3. FFM (kg) = 13.74 + 0.34 (HT^2/R) + 0.33 (BW) − 0.14 (age) + 6.18	Rising et al. (1991)
NIR (biceps)	Women (20-40 yr)	4. Db $(g/cc)^a$ = 1.02823066 − 0.080035 (ΔOD_2) − 0.000459 (age) − 0.000754 (BW) + 0.000493 (HT)	Heyward, Jenkins, et al. (1992)

Σ7SKF = sum of seven skinfolds (mm), HT = height (cm), R = resistance (Ω), BW = body weight (kg), ΔOD_2 = (OD_2 standard − OD_2 biceps).

[a] Use the following formula to convert Db to %BF: %BF = [(4.87/Db) − 4.41] × 100

it is probable that some Hispanics were included in these studies, cross-validation results for these equations were not reported specifically for this population.

Recently, we assessed the bone mineral content (BMC), bone mineral density (BMD), and total body water of 30 healthy, premenopausal (20 to 40 years of age) Hispanic women in New Mexico, using dual-energy x-ray absorptiometry (DXA) and deuterium dilution methods. The average body weight and relative body fat, as measured by hydrodensitometry and a four-component model, of this sample were 60.0 kg and 30.6 %BF. The average total body BMD, BMC, total body mineral (TBM), and total body water were, respectively, 1.161 g/cm^2, 2.41 kg, 3.08 kg, and 30.1 l. These values are close to those reported for white women (Hansen et al., 1993; Ortiz et al., 1992; Van Loan & Mayclin, 1992) with similar body weight (60 to 64 kg) and %BF (29% to 32%). Also, the relative mineral content of the FFB (7.4% FFB) was in agreement with the average value reported by Hansen et al. (1993) for premenopausal white women (7.3% FFB). Comparison of Siri's two-component model and Friedl's four-component model that adjusts body density (Db) for body mineral and body water yielded significantly different estimates of %BF for the Hispanic women in this sample (26.9% and 30.6%, respectively). These data suggest that the FFB density of Hispanic women is greater than the assumed value for the reference body (1.10 g/cc). In fact, the density of the FFB of Hispanic women in this sample was estimated to be 1.105 g/cc using a FFB-mineral content of 7.4% and FFB-water content of 72.8%.

Skinfold Equations for Hispanics

Generalized SKF equations (Jackson & Pollock, 1978; Jackson, Pollock, & Ward, 1980) have proven to be good predictors of Db in other racial groups (Hortobagyi, Israel, Houmard, McCammon, et al., 1992; McLean & Skinner, 1992; Paijmans, Wilmore, & Wilmore, 1992; Sparling et al., 1993) and are currently being used to assess the body composition of Hispanic individuals. Recently, we cross-validated Jackson's Σ3SKF and Σ7SKF equations for a sample of Hispanic women, 20 to 40 years of age (Heyward, Stolarczyk, et al., 1994). The Σ7SKF equation (Table 8.4) accurately estimated the average Db of this sample with an acceptable prediction error (E = 0.0078 g/cc). In contrast, the average Db was significantly overestimated using the Σ3SKF equation, and the total error was unacceptable (E = 0.0100 g/cc). Thus, *we recommend using the Σ7SKF equation to estimate the Db of young, healthy Hispanic women.* To convert Db to relative body fat (%BF), use the population-specific equation for Hispanic women (Table 8.4). Unfortunately, at this time, there are no research data to support the use of the SKF method for assessing the body composition of Hispanic men.

Bioelectrical Impedance Equations for Hispanics

Using samples of 42 Hispanic men and 30 Hispanic women from New Mexico, we cross-validated previously published BIA equations (Gray et al., 1989; Lohman, 1992; Rising et al., 1991; Segal et al., 1988; Van Loan & Mayclin, 1987). Total body density was assessed by hydrodensitometry and converted to relative body fat using Siri's two-component model equation. The total prediction errors of these equations ranged from 2.8 to 4.9 kg for men (Heyward, Wilson, & Stolarczyk, 1994) and 1.6 to 4.6 kg for women (Stolarczyk et al., 1995). It was interesting to note that all of these equations, with the exception of the Rising Pima Indian equation, significantly underestimated the average FFM of Hispanic men. Cross-validation of the Rising equation produced an acceptable prediction error (SEE = 3.4 kg) and closely estimated the average FFM of Hispanic men (63.4 vs. 63.3 kg).

As mentioned earlier, the Rising equation was developed using the Keys and Brozek (1953) two-component model conversion formula which systematically underestimates %BF in each individual. Therefore, it was surprising that this equation worked for Hispanic men in our sample, given that our reference values of FFM were derived from Siri's two-component model equation. One possible explanation is that the average FFM in the Hispanic men (63.2 kg) was almost identical to that of the Pima Indians (63.5 kg) used to develop Rising's equation. Also, the average age of both samples was similar (34 vs. 30 years of age, respectively, for Hispanics and Pima Indians). In addition, Samet et al. (1988) noted genetic similarities between Mexican Americans and American Indians. These findings suggest that future research needs to test the generalizability of race-specific equations developed for American Indian and Hispanic populations. Until new race-specific equations are developed for Hispanic men, *we recommend using Rising's BIA equation* (Table 8.4).

For Hispanic women, the Lohman, Gray, and Segal equations accurately predicted two-component model estimates of FFM within ±1 kg (Stolarczyk et al., 1995). The prediction errors for these equations were similar, ranging from 1.9 to 2.1 kg. Although any of these three BIA equations can be used to estimate FFM of Hispanic women, Gray's generalized equation (Table 8.4) is recommended for two reasons: (a) The Segal equations are fatness-specific; therefore, in order to select the appropriate equation, you must determine if your client's %BF is greater or less than 30 %BF, and (b) the Lohman equations are age-specific; therefore, two separate equations must be used to estimate FFM of women 18 to 29 years and 30 to 49 years.

Near-Infrared Interactance Equations for Hispanics

We do not recommend using the Futrex-5000 NIR manufacturer's equation for estimating body fat of Hispanic women and men. Cross-validation of this equation yielded an unacceptable prediction error (SEE = 6.4 %BF) and significantly underestimated the average body fat of our samples by 2.4 %BF (unpublished observations).

In addition, we cross-validated NIR equations developed for a multi-ethnic sample of women (86% white, 9% Hispanic, 4% American Indian, and 1% black) (Heyward, Jenkins, et al., 1992) and American Indian women (Hicks, Heyward, Flores, et al., 1993). Heyward's NIR equation accurately estimated the average body density of Hispanic women with an acceptable prediction error (E = 0.0081 g/cc). However, the Hick's NIR equation significantly underestimated the average Db of this sample, and the prediction error (E = 0.0093 g/cc) was large (Heyward, Stolarczyk, Goodman, et al., 1994). Based on these results, *we recommend using the Heyward NIR equation to estimate Db of young, Hispanic women.* To convert Db to %BF, use the race-specific conversion formula in Table 8.4.

Anthropometric Equations for Hispanics

As noted for other ethnic groups, there are no data supporting the use of the anthropometric method (circumference and bony diameter measures) to assess body composition of your Hispanic clients.

Assessing Body Composition of Asians

The Asian population is the largest population in the world and the second fastest growing minority population in the United States (U.S. Department of Commerce, 1991). Yet, there are no published race-specific body composition prediction equations that have been cross-validated for the U.S. Asian population. Recently, Wang et al. (1995) developed bioelectrical impedance equations for Asian Americans; however, these equations need to be cross-validated on additional samples of Asian American men and women.

The only published body composition prediction equations for Asian populations were developed for Japanese Natives using hydrodensitometry and two-component model reference measures. These equations should not be used to assess the body composition of Japanese Americans or individuals from other Asian populations. In this section, the FFB of Japanese Natives is described. Also, body composition methods and equations applicable to this population are presented in Table 8.5. In chapter 6, body composition equations for Japanese Native children were presented (Table 6.1).

Fat-Free Body Composition of Asians

Clearly, there is a lack of data describing the fat-free body composition of Asian populations. Although DeWaart, Li, and Deurenberg (1993) measured

Table 8.5 Prediction Equations for Japanese Natives

Method	Gender	Equation	Reference
SKF (*triceps + subscapular*)	Women (18-23 yr)	1. Db $(g/cc)^a$ = 1.0897 − 0.00133 (ΣSKF)	Nagamine & Suzuki (1964)
	Men (18-27 yr)	2. Db $(g/cc)^a$ = 1.0913 − 0.00116 (ΣSKF)	Nagamine & Suzuki (1964)
BIA	Women (18-54 yr)	3. Db $(g/cc)^a$ = 1.1628 − 0.1067 (BW × Z/HT^2)	Nakadomo et al. (1990)
	Obese women (18-68 yr) and (25-60 %BF)	4. Db $(g/cc)^a$ = 1.1307 − 0.0719 (BW × Z/HT^2) − 0.0003 (age)	Tanaka et al. (1992)
	Men (18-56 yr)	5. Db $(g/cc)^a$ = 1.1492 − 0.0918 (BW × Z/HT^2)	Nakadomo et al. (1990)

ΣSKF = sum of skinfolds (mm), BW = body weight (kg), Z = impedance (Ω), HT = height (cm)

[a]Use the following formulas to convert Db to %BF: Men (18-48 yr) %BF = [(4.97/Db) − 4.52] × 100; Women (18-48 yr) %BF = [(4.76/Db) − 4.28] × 100; Men (61-78 yr) %BF = [(4.87/Db) − 4.41] × 100; Women (61-78 yr) %BF = [(4.95/Db) − 4.50] × 100

total body water (TBW) to assess the body composition of Chinese women, they did not report the average TBW for their sample. Using the average TBW and FFM values reported by Wang et al. (1995), the relative hydration of the FFB was 77.3% and 78.3% for Asian men and women, respectively. These values indicate that the relative water content of the FFB of Asian Americans is greater than the assumed values for the reference body (73.8% FFB).

Based on average bone mineral content (BMC) values reported for younger, middle-aged, and older Japanese Native adults, we calculated an estimated total body mineral (BMC × 1.279) for each group. The relative mineral composition of the FFM was 8.6% for younger and middle-aged women and 6.6% for older women. Compared to other ethnic groups, the relative mineral content of the FFB in younger and middle-aged Japanese women is higher and reflects a smaller FFM (34 kg) and higher fat content (32 %BF and 36 %BF) for this population subgroup. For men, the respective values for younger, middle-aged, and older groups were 6.3%, 6.3%, and 7.4% FFM. Assuming a relative FFM hydration of 73%, the estimated density of the FFB is approximately 1.10 g/cc for men, 1.111 g/cc for younger and middle-aged women, and 1.105 g/cc for older women (Table 1.6). It is important to note that these estimates of FFB composition are based on data from an extremely small number of individuals (~11 men and ~11 women per age group). Therefore, the FFB constants may not be representative of this population, and the race-specific conversion formulas derived from these estimates of FFB composition may need to be modified when more data become available in the future.

Skinfold Equations for Asians

Recently, Wang et al. (1994) developed SKF prediction equations for Asian American men (N = 110) and women (N = 132), ages 18 to 98 years. The sample was 93% Chinese, 4% Japanese, 2.5% Korean, and 1% Filipino; 97% of this sample was born in Asia. These equations used body mass index, age, and four SKF measures to estimate %BF, measured by dual-photon absorptiometry. Although the prediction errors for these equations were fairly good (SEE = 3.5 %BF for women and 3.7 %BF for men), they still need to be cross-validated on additional samples of Asian men and women before we can recommend using them.

In addition, Wang et al. (1994) cross-validated the Durnin and Womersley (Σ4SKF) and Jackson (Σ3SKF) equations. Both equations significantly underestimated the average %BF of Asian women and men by 1 %BF to 2.9 %BF, and the prediction errors were large (SEE = 4.0 %BF to 4.3 %BF). They attributed these findings to differences in fat distribution between Asian and white populations. Asians had significantly larger biceps, abdomen, suprailiac, and subscapular SKF measurements compared to white men and women in their study.

Nagamine and Suzuki (1964) developed gender-specific SKF equations for young, Japanese Native adults (18 to 27 years of age) using hydrodensitometry as the reference method. These equations accurately estimated (SEE = 3.7 %BF) the body composition of Japanese Native men (18 to 56 years of age) but underestimated the average body fatness of Japanese Native women (18 to 54 years) by 3 %BF (SEE = 4.3 %BF) (Nakadomo, Tanaka, Hazama, & Maeda, 1990). Also, the equation had only a fair degree of accuracy when it was applied to a sample of obese, Japanese women (Tanaka et al., 1992). However, other researchers reported that these equations accurately predicted body fat (SEE = 3.4 %BF) in Japanese Native adults (Sawai, Mutoh, & Miyashita, 1990). *Therefore, we recommend using these equations along with the appropriate race-specific conversion formula (Table 8.5) to assess body fatness in this population.*

Bioelectrical Impedance Equations for Asians

Nakadomo et al. (1990) cross-validated the BIA equations of Segal et al. (1988) and Lukaski et al. (1986) for Japanese Natives. Both equations systematically overestimated the average FFM of Japanese men and women by 3 to 4 kg. Thus, they developed gender-specific BIA equations, with acceptable prediction errors (1.9 and 2.2 kg FFM, respectively, for men and women). However, this equation failed to accurately estimate the body composition of obese, Japanese women (SEE = 0.0089 g/cc or ~4 %BF) (Tanaka et al., 1992). Consequently, Tanaka and associates developed and cross-validated a fat-specific BIA equation for obese, Japanese Native women (Table 8.5).

Near-Infrared Interactance Equations for Asians

Like other ethnic groups, there is a lack of research substantiating the validity for the NIR method for assessing body composition in Asian Americans and Japanese Natives. We obtained one abstract (from Futrex) that was translated from Japanese to English and reprinted from the annals of Tokyo University (Sawai et al., 1990). These researchers found no significant difference between %BF estimated from the Futrex-5000 NIR equation and hydrodensitometry (SEE = 3.3 %BF) for Japanese men and women. Because we cannot verify the accuracy of this translation or provide a complete citation for this work, it may be better to use alternative methods to assess body composition of Japanese Native adults.

Anthropometric Equations for Asians

Although Nagamine and Suzuki (1964) measured circumferences and skeletal diameters of Japanese Natives and compared these values to those reported for men and women in the United States, they did not develop anthropometric equations for this population. Therefore, alernative methods, like skinfold and bioelectrical impedance, can be used instead.

Assessing Body Composition of Whites

A vast amount of research has focused on quantifying the fat-free body composition of white men and women and on developing methods and equations for estimating body fatness in this population. In this section, body composition methods applicable to this ethnic group are presented, and prediction equations are summarized in Table 8.6.

Fat-Free Body Composition of Whites

As discussed in chapter 6, the composition and overall density of the FFB increases from childhood to adulthood for both females and males. The average FFB density of white females at any age is somewhat less than that of males due to the relatively greater hydration of their FFB (Lohman, 1986). The FFB density of younger and middle-aged men, estimated from multicomponent models, is remarkably similar to the assumed value (1.10 g/cc) of Siri's (1961) two-component model. Therefore, many prediction equations based on two-component model estimates of body composition work quite well in this population subgroup.

On the other hand, the average FFB density in younger and middle-aged women (1.097 g/cc) is somewhat less; thus, the Siri two-component model systematically overestimates average body fatness in white women. Because there is much interindividual variability in FFB composition (Table 1.5), experts recommend using multicomponent models to develop prediction equations, especially for white women. Further research is needed to establish the water and mineral content of the FFB for white women.

Skinfold Equations for Whites

Although there are many age-specific SKF equations for white men (Lohman 1992; Sloan, 1967), there is an abundance of research demonstrating the applicability of Jackson and Pollock's (1978) generalized SKF equations for this population subgroup. Cross-validation of these equations indicates prediction errors ranging from 2.6 %BF to 3.5 %BF for the Σ3SKF equation

Table 8.6 Prediction Equations for Whites

Method	Gender	Equation	Reference
SKF			
(*triceps + suprailiac + thigh*)	Women (18-55 yr)	1. Db (g/cc)^a = 1.0994921 − 0.0009929 ($\sum$3SKF) + 0.0000023 ($\sum$3SKF)^2 − 0.0001392 (age)	Jackson et al. (1980)
(*chest + abdomen + thigh*)	Men (18-61 yr)	2. Db (g/cc)^a = 1.109380 − 0.0008267 ($\sum$3SKF) + 0.0000016 ($\sum$3SKF)^2 − 0.0002574 (age)	Jackson & Pollock (1978)
BIA	Women		
	(18-29 yr)	3. FFM (kg) = 0.476 (HT^2/R) + 0.295 (BW) + 5.49	Lohman (1992)
	(30-49 yr)	4. FFM (kg) = 0.493 (HT^2/R) + 0.141 (BW) + 11.59	Lohman (1992)
	(50-70 yr)	5. FFM (kg) = 0.474 (HT^2/R) + 0.180 (BW) + 7.3	Lohman (1992)
	(18-64 yr)	6. FFM (kg) = 0.00085 (HT^2) − 0.02375 (R) + 0.3736 (BW) − 0.1531 (age) + 13.4947	Van Loan & Mayclin (1987)
	(22-74 yr)	7. FFM (kg) = 0.00151 (HT^2) − 0.0344 (R) + 0.140 (BW) − 0.158 (age) + 20.387	Gray et al. (1989)

(continued)

Table 8.6 (*continued*)

Method	Gender	Equation	Reference
BIA (*continued*)	Men (18–29 yr) (<20 %BF) (17–62 yr)	8. FFM (kg) = 0.485 (HT^2/R) + 0.338 (BW) + 5.32	Lohman (1992)
		9. FFM (kg) = 0.00066360 (HT^2) − 0.02117 (R) + 0.62854 (BW) − 0.12380 (age) + 9.33285	Segal et al. (1988)
	(≥20 %BF) (17–62 yr)	10. FFM (kg) = 0.00088580 (HT^2) − 0.02999 (R) + 0.42688 (BW) − 0.07002 (age) + 14.52435	Segal et al. (1988)
NIR (*biceps*)	Women (20–72 yr)	11. Db (g/cc)[a] = 1.02823066 − 0.080035 (ΔOD_2) − 0.000459 (age) − 0.000754 (BW) + 0.000493 (HT)	Heyward, Jenkins et al. (1992)
Anthropometry	Women (15–79 yr)	12. Db (g/cc)[a] = 1.168297 − 0.002824 (AB C) + 0.0000122098 $(AB\ C)^2$ − 0.000733128 (hip C) + 0.000510477 (HT) − 0.000216161 (age)	Tran & Weltman (1989)
	Men (18–40 yr)	13. FFM (kg) = 39.652 + 1.0932 (BW) + 0.8370 (bi-iliac D) + 0.3297 $(AB_1\ C)$ − 1.0008 $(AB_2\ C)$ − 0.6478 (knee C)	Wilmore & Behnke (1969)

Σ3SKF = sum of three skinfolds (mm); HT = height (cm); R = resistance (Ω); BW = body weight (kg); ΔOD_2 = (OD_2 standard − OD_2 biceps); C = circumference (cm), AB C (cm): average abdominal circumference = $[(AB_1 + AB_2)/2]$, where AB_1 (cm) = abdominal circumference anteriorly midway between the xiphoid process of sternum and the umbilicus and laterally between the lower end of the rib cage and iliac crests, and AB_2 (cm) = abdominal circumference at the umbilicus level; D = diameter (cm)

[a]Use the following formulas to convert Db to %BF: Men %BF = [(4.95/Db) − 4.50] × 100, Women %BF = [(5.01/Db) − 4.57] × 100

(McLean & Skinner, 1992; Paijmans et al., 1992) and the Σ7SKF equation (Hortobagyi, Israel, Houmard, McCammon, et al., 1992; Israel et al., 1989; Jackson et al., 1988). Typically, there are small differences (up to 1.4 %BF) between measured and SKF-predicted body fat in these samples.

In contrast, one study reported that the Σ3SKF equation significantly underestimated average %BF of white men, 22 to 75 years of age (Clark, Kuta, & Sullivan, 1993). However, some of their subjects were older (> 61 years) and obese (up to 30 %BF). Wilmore, McBride, and Wilmore (1994) reported that the Σ7SKF equation significantly underestimated the average %BF of overweight and obese men by 4 %BF, with a prediction error (SEE) of 4.1 %BF. Jackson and Pollock (1985) warned that these equations may not be accurate for estimating %BF of men whose Σ3SKF (chest, abdomen, and thigh SKFs) exceeds 118 mm.

The Jackson, Pollock, and Ward (1980) generalized SKF equations also show good predictive accuracy (SEE = 2.9 %BF to 3.5 %BF) and small differences (0.3 %BF to 1.3 %BF) when they are used to estimate the body fatness of white women (Eaton, Israel, O'Brien, Hortobagyi, & McCammon, 1993; Heyward, Cook, et al., 1992; Jackson et al., 1988; McLean & Skinner, 1992). As mentioned for men, these equations generally work best when they are applied to nonobese women. Wilmore, McBride, and Wilmore (1994) noted that average %BF of overweight and obese women was significantly underestimated by 2.8 %BF using the Jackson Σ7SKF equation. We found that the Jackson Σ3SKF equation significantly underestimated the average body fat of obese women by 3.7 %BF (Heyward, Cook, et al., 1992). Likewise, Paijmans et al. (1992) reported that the average body fatness of obese, white women and men was underestimated by 5.5 %BF.

Based on these studies, you may *use either the Σ3SKF or Σ7SKF equation to estimate Db of white men and women.* However, for practical purposes, we recommend using the Σ3SKF equation (Table 8.6). To convert Db to %BF, use the conversion formulas presented in Table 8.6.

Bioelectrical Impedance Equations for Whites

For the BIA method, there are many age-specific and generalized equations that are applicable to the white adult population. Some of these equations (Lohman, 1992; Lukaski et al., 1986) are programmed into your BIA analyzer. As a reminder, before using your analyzer, you need to find out which equations the manufacturer has programmed into the software version accompanying it. The overwhelming majority of BIA equations are derived from two-component models. Therefore, these equations may systematically underestimate the FFM in white women. We found only two BIA equations based on multicomponent body composition models (Lohman, 1992; Van Loan et al., 1990). Lohman's age-specific equation for 50- to 70-year-old women adjusts for changes in bone mineral with aging; Van Loan's equation accounts for interindividual differences in total body water. However, this equation was not cross-validated in their study.

Lohman's (1992) age-specific BIA equations accurately estimated average FFM of younger (18-30 years) and older (50-70 years) white women. The prediction errors for these equations were 2.0 to 2.8 kg or < 3.5 %BF, and the difference between reference and predicted body fat was less than 1 %BF (Graves, Pollock, Calvin, Van Loan, & Lohman, 1989; Jenkins et al., 1994). For women from 30 to 50 years of age, we found a small systematic underestimation of average FFM using Lohman's equation (Wilson et al., 1992). Lohman's equation for younger women (18-30 years) grossly under-estimated the body fat of obese, white women by 7 %BF on average (Hey-ward, Cook, et al., 1992), suggesting that equations developed specifically for obese women need to be used (see chapter 9).

As an alternative to Lohman's age-specific equations, the Segal et al. (1988) fat-specific equations or the generalized BIA equations of Gray et al. (1989) or Van Loan and Mayclin (1987) may be used (SEE = 1.8 to 3.1 kg) to estimate the FFM of white women (Gray et al., 1989; Jenkins et al., 1994). One shortcoming of Segal's fat-specific equations is that the client needs to be classified as nonobese (< 30 %BF) or obese (≥ 30 %BF) in order to select the appropriate equation. To do this, Segal recommends measuring the sum of four skinfolds, but, this negates the advantage of using BIA as a simple method requiring less technician skill than the SKF method. As an alternative, generalized equations, applicable to white women varying greatly in age (22 to 74 years of age for the Gray equation and 18 to 64 years of age for the Van Loan and Mayclin equation) and level of body fatness (19% to 59% for the Gray equation), can be used.

Overall, *we recommend using either Lohman's (1992) age-specific equations or the generalized equations of Gray et al. (1989) and Van Loan and Mayclin (1987) to assess body composition of white women.* These equations are presented in Table 8.6 and summarized in the Quick Reference Guide in Appendix A. Cross-validation studies indicate large prediction errors (SEE = 3.6 %BF to 5.0 %BF) for the Deurenberg et al. (1990), Lukaski et al. (1986), and Segal et al. (1985) BIA equations (Graves et al., 1989; Jackson et al., 1988; Jenkins et al., 1994; Van Loan & Mayclin, 1987). Based on these findings, we suggest that you do not use these equations to estimate body composition of white women.

Similarly, the BIA equations of Lukaski et al. (1986), Segal et al. (1985), and Deurenberg, van der Kooy, Leenan, Westrate, and Seidell (1991) do not appear to be applicable for adult, white men (SEE = 3.8 %BF to 5.0 %BF), as they typically underestimate the average FFM by 2 to 5 kg (Eckerson, Housh, & Johnson, 1992; Graves et al., 1989; Jackson et al., 1988; Pierson et al., 1991; Van Loan & Mayclin, 1987). This is especially true for lean men with body fat levels ranging between 3 %BF and 13 %BF (Eckerson et al., 1992).

In comparison, Lohman's (1992) age-specific (18 to 30 years) equation and Segal's et al. (1988) fatness-specific equations have smaller prediction errors

(SEE = 1.8 to 3.1 kg) (Eckerson et al., 1992; Gray et al., 1989). Therefore, we recommend using these equations to estimate FFM of men (Table 8.6). However, to use Segal's fat-specific equations you need to select the appropriate formula (< 20 %BF or ≥ 20 %BF) beforehand by visually assessing your client's body fat level. This is not a problem for very lean or obese men. If you are uncertain about your client's body fat level, you need to measure the sum of four skinfolds (biceps + triceps + subscapular + suprailiac). When your client's sum of four skinfolds (Σ4SKF) exceeds 54 mm for 17 to 29 years, 43 mm for 30 to 39 years, 37 mm for 40 to 49 years, or 33 mm for 50+ years, you should use the ≥ 20 %BF equation. Alternatively, for younger men, 18 to 30 years of age, Lohman's (1992) age-specific BIA equation can be used.

Near-Infrared Interactance Equations for Whites

As discussed in chapter 4, there are many questions concerning the use of the NIR method to assess body composition. Much of the NIR research has focused on the validity of the Futrex-5000 manufacturer's equation for estimating body fat of white men and women. Regardless of gender, the prediction error of the manufacturer's equation in the white population is unacceptable with standard errors of estimate (SEEs) ranging from 3.1 %BF to 4.8 %BF for men and 3.7 %BF to 5.8 %BF for women (Eaton et al., 1993; Elia, Parkinson, & Diaz, 1990; Heyward, Jenkins, et al., 1992; Israel et al., 1989; McLean & Skinner, 1992; Nielsen et al., 1992). Based on data from nine studies, this equation underestimated the body fat in nonobese, white adults by an average of 2.5 %BF (0.9% to 6.0 %BF). Therefore, *we do not recommend using the %BF estimates from your Futrex-5000 analyzer.*

To our knowledge, there is only one other published NIR equation (Heyward, Jenkins, et al., 1992). We developed this equation using a predominantly white sample (85%) of women, ages 20 to 72 years. The prediction error (SEE = 0.0082 g/cc or 3.6 %BF) for this equation is good, but additional cross-validation studies are needed to evaluate the extent of its applicability to other samples of white women. In the meantime, we suggest using this equation (Table 8.6) to assess the Db of your white, female clients only when other methods, such as SKF and BIA, are unavailable to you. To convert Db to %BF, use the conversion formula for white women, 20 to 80 years of age (Table 8.6).

Anthropometric Equations for Whites

Wilmore and Behnke (1969, 1970) developed age-specific anthropometric equations to estimate body density and lean body mass (LBM) of young women and men using combinations of skeletal diameter and circumference measures. Cross-validation of the equations indicated that the male equation overestimated LBM by 1.8 kg (SEE = 2.5 kg). The accuracy of these equations was generally poorer (SEE = 3.0 kg) for women than for men (Katch & McArdle, 1973).

As an alternative, we recommend a generalized, anthropometric equation to estimate the Db of white women, 15 to 79 years of age (Tran & Weltman, 1989). This equation has good predictive accuracy (SEE = 0.0082 g/cc or 3.6 %BF) in this population. On the other hand, the generalized anthropometric equation developed for white men (21 to 78 years) should not be used because of its large prediction error (SEE = 4.4 %BF) (Tran & Weltman, 1988). Selected anthropometric equations are presented in Table 8.6 and in the Quick Reference Guide. Additional anthropometric equations applicable to obese white adults are included in chapter 9.

KEY POINTS

▮ Obesity is a serious problem in some minority populations. American Indian women and men, as well as black and Hispanic women, have been targeted for weight loss.

▮ The FFB density of American Indians and blacks is greater than that of whites, primarily due to their higher bone mineral content and bone density.

▮ There are race-specific SKF, BIA, and NIR equations to estimate the body composition of American Indian women.

▮ The skinfold method (Jackson generalized Σ7SKF) can be used to estimate body density of black men and women.

▮ Selected SKF, BIA, and NIR equations can be used to estimate body composition of Hispanic women.

▮ Race-specific SKF and BIA equations have been developed for the Japanese Native population; however, race-specific equations developed for Asian American populations need to be cross-validated.

▮ The body composition of whites can be assessed using selected SKF, BIA, NIR, and anthropometric equations.

Chapter 9

Body Composition and Levels of Body Fatness

In chapter 1, we presented the concept that individuals may be at-risk for disease if relative body fat is too high (≥ 25 %BF and ≥ 32 %BF, respectively, for men and women) or too low (< 5 %BF and < 8 %BF to 12 %BF, respectively, for men and women). Regardless of age, gender, and ethnicity, body fatness is a critical component of the individual's health profile. Thus, health and fitness professionals need to be able to identify underfat and obese individuals and to calculate body weights that correspond to fatness levels that are optimal for good health.

As mentioned throughout this book, individuals who are overweight or obese have increased risk of cardiovascular disease, hypertension, Type II diabetes, hyperlipidemia, obstructive pulmonary disease, osteoarthritis, and certain types of cancers (National Institutes of Health, 1985). At the opposite extreme, individuals with too little body fat tend to be malnourished, and, therefore, may have a relatively higher risk of fluid-electrolyte imbalances, osteoporosis and osteopenia, bone fractures, muscle wasting, cardiac arrythmias and sudden death, peripheral edema, as well as renal and reproductive disorders (Fohlin, 1977; Mazess, Barden, & Ohlrich, 1990; Vaisman, Corey, Rossi, Goldberg, & Pencharz, 1988).

One disease associated with extremely low body fat levels is anorexia nervosa. Anorexia nervosa is an eating disorder found primarily in females and is characterized by excessive weight loss. The prevalence of anorexia nervosa is estimated at 1% of the general female population (American Psychiatric Association, 1994). Compared to normal women, anorexics have extremely low body fat (7.7 %BF to 13 %BF), increased total body water due to an expanded extracellular water volume (32% of body weight), some signs of muscle wasting (average fat-free mass = 39 kg), and less bone mineral content and bone density (1.92 kg and 0.99 g/cm^2, respectively) (Dempsey et al., 1984; Mazess, Barden, & Ohlrich, 1990; Vaisman, Rossi, et al., 1988). Mazess, Barden, & Ohlrich (1990) reported that the average bone mineral density of the spine of 18- to 27-year-old anorexic women was equivalent to that of 70-year-old women.

In this chapter, methods and prediction equations suitable for estimating the body composition of underfat and obese individuals are presented (Tables 9.1 and 9.2). These equations are also summarized in the Quick Reference Guide in Appendix A. To assess the body composition of anorexic women, the skinfold method is recommended. For obese men and women, either the bioelectrical impedance or anthropometric methods may be used.

Assessing Body Composition of Anorexic Females

Changes in water, bone, and muscle associated with anorexia nervosa will affect the FFB composition and estimation of body fat from total body density. Based on data reported in the literature, we estimated the FFB components and their corresponding densities (d) to be 76% water (d = 0.9937 g/cc) (Dempsey et al., 1984), 6.3% mineral (d = 2.73 g/cc) (Mazess, Barden, & Ohlrich, 1990), and 17.7% protein (d = 1.34 g/cc), yielding a FFB density of only 1.087 g/cc for anorexic women. Based on this FFB density, we derived the following formula for estimating %BF from Db: %BF = (5.26/Db − 4.83) × 100. Compared to this formula, the average body fatness of anorexic women will be systematically overestimated by 3 %BF to 4 %BF when two-component model equations (Siri, 1961; Brozek et al., 1963) are used to estimate %BF from Db. Thus, we recommend using the derived population-specific conversion formula to assess the relative body fatness of anorexic women.

To date there are no skinfold (SKF), bioelectrical impedance (BIA), near-infrared interactance (NIR), or anthropometric equations developed specifically for anorexic females. Vaisman, Rossi, et al. (1988) assessed the body composition of anorexic girls, ages 13 to 17 years, using the SKF equation developed by Durnin and Rahaman (1967). The average body fat of their sample (17 %BF) was most likely overestimated given that Siri's two-component model formula was used to convert body density to relative body fat. Using the conversion formula we derived based on multicomponent model estimates of total body water and body mineral, we estimated the average body fatness of their sample to be considerably lower (13 %BF).

Therefore, until additional research and prediction equations based on multicomponent models are developed, we suggest using the generalized SKF equations of Jackson et al. (1980) to predict Db and the population-specific conversion formula (Table 9.1) to estimate relative body fatness of anorexic women. The BIA method is not recommended given that the relative hydration of the FFB and the ratio of extracellular to intracellular water are abnormally high in anorexic women (Vaisman, Rossi, et al., 1988).

Assessing Body Composition of Obese

Changes in water, skeletal muscle, and bone mass associated with obesity affect the composition and density of the fat-free body (FFB) and the estimates of relative body fat (%BF) from Db. Research indicates that the relative hydration of the FFB increases with body fatness. Hydration levels in obese men (74.2% FFB) and women (76% to 77% FFB) are higher than those of leaner men (72.6% FFB) and women (73% to 74% FFB) (Albu et al., 1989; Segal, Wang, Gutin, Pierson, & Van Itallie, 1987). The increase in total body water (TBW) with obesity is not proportionately distributed between the extracellular and intracellular fluid compartments. Waki et al. (1991) noted a relatively greater increase in extracellular water compared to intracellular water in obese women. These researchers suggested that two-component body composition models, based on assumptions that water distribution is constant and independent of body fatness, are likely to result in larger-than-expected errors in estimating the body composition of some obese individuals.

In fact, Deurenberg, Leenan, van der Kooy, and Hautvast (1989) demonstrated that the Siri two-component model overestimates the average relative body fat (%BF) of obese individuals by 2 %BF to 4 %BF. Assuming an increase in relative body water and decreases in relative body mineral and protein, they estimated the FFB density to be 1.0929 g/cc and derived the following fatness-specific formula for converting Db to %BF in obese individuals: %BF = [(5.10/Db) − 4.67] × 100.

In addition to greater hydration of the FFB, obese individuals tend to have increased bone mass and relative total body mineral (TBM), thereby countering the effect of TBW on FFB density to some extent. Lindsay, Cosman, Herrington, and Himmelstein (1992) noted that the total body bone mineral (TBBM) of obese (> 33 %BF) women was significantly greater than that of leaner (< 33 %BF) women. Also, the relative TBBM (TBBM/FFM) was higher in premenopausal, obese women. Based on these data, we estimated the relative TBM to be 8% FFM in obese women. This value was similar to that reported (8.1% FFM) for a sample of obese, American Indian women with an average body fat of 37% (Stolarczyk et al., 1994).

Table 9.1 Prediction Equation for Anorexic Women

Method	Gender	Equation	Reference
SKF (*triceps + suprailiac + thigh*)	Women (18-55 yr)	1. Db (g/cc)[a] = $1.0994921 - 0.0009929\ (\Sigma 3SKF) + 0.0000023\ (\Sigma 3SKF)^2 - 0.0001392$ (age)	Jackson et al. (1980)

$\Sigma 3SKF$ = sum of three skinfolds (mm)

[a]Use the following formula to convert Db to %BF: %BF = $[(5.26/Db) - 4.83] \times 100$

Table 9.2 Prediction Equations for Obese Individuals

Method	Gender	Equation	Reference
BIA	Women (19-59 %BF)	1. FFM (kg) = $0.00151\ (HT^2) - 0.0344\ (R) + 0.140\ (BW) - 0.158$ (age) $+ 20.387$	Gray et al. (1989)
	Men (9-45 %BF)	2. FFM (kg) = $0.00139\ (HT^2) - 0.0801\ (R) + 0.187\ (BW) + 39.830$	Gray et al. (1989)
Anthropometry	Women (20-60 yr)	3. %BF = $0.11077\ (AB\ C) - 0.17666\ (HT) + 0.14354\ (BW) + 51.03301$	Weltman et al. (1988)
	Men (24-68 yr)	4. %BF = $0.31457\ (AB\ C) - 0.10969\ (BW) + 10.8336$	Weltman et al. (1987)

HT = height (cm); R = resistance (Ω); BW = body weight (kg); AB C (cm): average abdominal circumference = $[(AB_1 + AB_2)/2]$, where AB_1 (cm) = abdominal circumference anteriorly midway between the xyphoid process of the sternum and the umbilicus and laterally between the lower end of the rib cage and iliac crests, and AB_2 (cm) = abdominal circumference at the umbilicus level

Assuming that the FFB composition of obese women is 76% water (Albu et al., 1989; Segal et al., 1987), 8% mineral (Lindsay et al., 1992), and 16% protein, we estimated the FFB density of this group to be 1.0983 g/cc, which is slightly higher than the value (1.0929 g/cc) theoretically derived by Deurenberg, Leenan, van der Kooy, and Hautvast (1989). Using our estimate of FFB density, the following fatness-specific conversion formula was calculated for obese women: %BF = [(5.00/Db) − 4.56] × 100.

Skinfold Equations for Obese

A number of investigators have tested the accuracy of population-specific (Durnin & Womersley, 1974) and generalized (Jackson & Pollock, 1978; Jackson et al., 1980) skinfold (SKF) equations in overweight and obese samples. Overall, it appears that the SKF method and these equations have limited applicability to obese individuals.

Although some obese individuals were included in the original samples used to develop Jackson's generalized SKF equations, Jackson and Pollock (1985) warned that these equations may produce larger than expected prediction errors when they are applied to individuals whose sum of seven skinfolds (Σ7SKF) exceeds 266 mm for women and 272 mm for men. In fact, the Σ3SKF, Σ4SKF, and Σ7SKF equations significantly underestimated the average relative body fat of obese men and women by 1.5 %BF to 4 %BF (Gray et al., 1990; Heyward, Cook, et al., 1992; Teran et al., 1991; Wilmore, McBride, & Wilmore, 1994). Also, the prediction errors for these equations were high, with standard errors of estimate ranging from 3.4 %BF to 5.1 %BF.

In general, similar results were observed for Durnin and Womersley's (1974) population-specific SKF equations. Although it has been reported that these equations significantly overestimate the average %BF of overweight and obese men and women by 3 %BF to 4 %BF (Wilmore, McBride, & Wilmore, 1994), other researchers have found that these equations underestimate relative body fat in obese samples by 1.5 %BF to 12 %BF, with SEEs ranging from 3.4 %BF to 7 %BF (Elia et al., 1990; Fulcher et al., 1991; Gray et al., 1990; Teran et al., 1991). However, in one study of slightly obese men, the Durnin and Womersley equations accurately estimated their average body fatness before weight loss (SEE = 3.5 %BF) (Ross, Leger, Martin, & Roy, 1989). This discrepancy among studies most likely reflects differences in the level of body fatness between samples.

Overall, *experts agree that the SKF method should not be used to estimate the body composition of obese individuals.* With increasing levels of body fatness, the proportion of subcutaneous to total body fat changes, thereby affecting the relationship between the ΣSKF and total body density. Furthermore, the applicability of the SKF method in obese individuals is limited for the following reasons:

1. Site selection and palpation of bony landmarks are more difficult in obese individuals (Bray & Gray, 1988a).
2. The SKF thickness may be larger than the jaw aperature of most calipers, and it may not be possible to lift the SKF from the underlying tissue in some obese clients (Gray et al., 1990).
3. There is greater variation in the depth at which the caliper tips can be placed on the SKF, and the caliper tips may slide on larger SKFs.
4. Variability in adipose tissue composition may affect SKF compressibility in obese clients (Clarys, Martin, Drinkwater, & Marfell-Jones, 1987).
5. There is greater variability among testers when measuring larger SKF thicknesses (Bray & Gray, 1988a).

In short, these factors limit the accuracy and precision of SKF measurements in obese individuals. Therefore, *we do not recommend using the SKF method to assess the body composition of your obese clients.*

Bioelectrical Impedance Equations for Obese

Unlike the SKF method, bioelectrical impedance (BIA) appears to be a promising method for assessing body composition of obese individuals, provided that BIA equations developed specifically for obese populations are selected for this purpose. The first fatness-specific BIA equations were developed by Segal et al. (1988) for women (< 30 %BF and ≥ 30 %BF) and men (< 20 %BF and ≥ 20 %BF). Cross-validation of the equations for obese men and women yielded smaller prediction errors (SEE = 2.8 and 2.0 kg, respectively) compared to generalized BIA equations (SEE = 3.6 and 2.4 kg, respectively), indicating that fatness-specific equations are more accurate in this population. In addition, other researchers have reported that Segal's fatness-specific equations accurately predicted two-component model estimates of average fat-free mass in obese, American Indian women (SEE = 2.7 kg), obese, white women (SEE = 2.4 kg), slightly obese men (SEE = 3.2 kg), and obese women and men with less than 42 %BF (SEE = 3.5 kg) (Gray et al., 1989; Jenkins et al., 1994; Ross et al., 1989; Stolarczyk et al., 1994).

However, Gray et al. (1989, 1990) noted that Segal's fatness-specific equations tended to systematically overestimate FFM in more obese men and women, especially for women whose relative body fat exceeded 48 %BF. As a result, Gray et al. (1989) developed generalized equations for men (9 %BF to 45 %BF) and women (19 %BF to 59 %BF) and a fatness-specific equation for very obese women (> 48 %BF). Although these equations were not cross-validated in their original study, we found that Gray's generalized equation for women accurately predicted two-component model estimates of FFM in white women (11 %BF to 58 %BF) and American Indian women (14 %BF to 54 %BF) (Jenkins et al., 1994; Stolarczyk et al., 1994). However, we were not able to cross-validate Gray's fatness-specific (> 48 %BF) equation because of the relatively small number of severely obese women in our sample.

Based on these studies, *we recommend using either Segal's fatness-specific (≥ 20 %BF for men and ≥ 30 %BF for women) equations, or Gray's generalized equations to assess the body composition of your obese clients.* However, we prefer Gray's equations (Table 9.2) because, to use Segal's equations, you will need to either visually determine that your client is obese or measure the sum of four skinfolds (Σ4SKF), as described in chapter 8. We do not recommend using the manufacturers' equations programmed in the software accompanying your BIA analyzers (Holtain, RJL, and Valhalla). Research clearly demonstrates that these equations systematically overestimate average FFM in obese women and men (Fulcher et al., 1991; Heyward, Cook, et al., 1992; Hodgdon & Fitzgerald, 1987; Ross et al., 1989; Segal et al., 1988).

Near-Infrared Interactance Equations for Obese

There is much evidence indicating that the near-infrared interactance (NIR) method and Futrex-5000 manufacturer's equation should not be used to assess body composition of obese individuals. In obese samples, this equation has large, unacceptable prediction errors (SEE = 3.8 %BF to 4.3 %BF) and systematically underestimates relative body fat by as much as 10 %BF to 16 %BF (Davis, Van Loan, Holly, Krstich, & Phinney, 1989; Elia et al., 1990; Heyward, Cook et al., 1992; Wilmore, McBride, & Wilmore, 1994). It appears that fat layering, which is characteristic of obese individuals with large amounts of subcutaneous fat, may affect the depth to which the near-infrared light penetrates the tissues at the measurement site. Quatrochi et al. (1992) reported that the relationship between optical density (OD) and SKF measures at the biceps site was stronger in leaner women (22 %BF) compared to obese women (39 %BF). This observation may explain why the degree of underestimation of %BF is markedly increased in more obese individuals (Davis et al., 1989; Elia et al., 1990).

Anthropometric Equations for Obese

In addition to bioelectrical impedance (BIA), anthropometric methods and equations appear to be suitable alternatives for assessing body composition of obese individuals. The advantages of using this method are:

a. It is less expensive than BIA and does not require the client to adhere to strict pretesting guidelines.
b. Compared to skinfolds, circumferences can be easily measured, regardless of the client's level of body fatness.

Weltman, Seip, and Tran (1987) developed an anthropometric equation to predict the fat-free mass (FFM) of obese (30 %BF to 45 %BF) men, 24 to 68 years of age, using abdominal circumferences and body weight as predictors.

Cross-validation of this equation yielded accurate estimates of average FFM and acceptable prediction error (SEE = 2.6 kg). In a similar study (Weltman et al., 1988) of obese women, cross-validation of the anthropometric equation predicting FFM indicated that this equation had only fair predictive accuracy (SEE = 3.2 kg). However, the accuracy of the equation estimating relative body fat in this sample was acceptable (SEE = 3.5 %BF).

Although Teran et al. (1991) developed anthropometric equations to estimate the relative body fatness of obese women, these equations had unacceptable prediction errors (SEE = 3.9 %BF to 4.3 %BF). The predictor variables in these equations include log transformations of skinfold and circumference measures, as well as residual lung volume, making them impractical for field and clinical use.

In summary, *we recommend using Weltman's (1987, 1988) fat-specific anthropometric equations to assess body composition of your obese clients.* These equations are presented in Table 9.2 and in the Quick Reference Guide in Appendix A.

KEY POINTS

▌ Men and women who are underfat (< 5 %BF and < 8 %BF to 12 %BF, respectively) or obese (≥ 25 %BF and ≥ 32 %BF, respectively) have a greater risk of disease.

▌ The FFB density of women with anorexia nervosa is less than 1.10 g/cc, resulting in a systematic overestimation of %BF when two-component body composition models and equations are used.

▌ There are no SKF, BIA, or anthropometric equations developed specifically for anorexic females.

▌ The FFB density of obese individuals is less than 1.10 g/cc, resulting in a systematic overestimation of %BF when two-component body composition models and equations are used.

▌ SKF and NIR methods are not recommended for assessing body composition of obese clients.

▌ Fatness-specific BIA and anthropometric equations can be used to assess body composition of obese clients.

Chapter *10*

Body Composition and Athletes

Body composition of athletic populations has been an interest of exercise scientists and clinicians specializing in sports medicine. Generally, a relatively low body fat is desirable to optimize physical performance in sports requiring jumping and running. A large muscle mass enhances performance in strength and power activities. For years, exercise scientists and sports medicine professionals have examined the physiological profiles of elite athletes. Typically, athletes and physically active individuals are leaner than sedentary individuals, regardless of gender. However, female athletes have relatively greater body fat than male athletes in a given sport, and the average body fatness depends on the type of sport and the athlete's position (Wilmore, 1983).

In addition to establishing physiological profiles, you can use body composition information to estimate the athlete's optimal body weight or competitive weight class for certain sports, such as wrestling and bodybuilding. *For males, experts agree that the minimal body fatness should not be less than 5 %BF* because some body fat is needed for normal physiological and metabolic functions. Likewise, the American College of Sports Medicine (1985) recommends using 5 %BF to determine the minimal body weight of wrestlers.

In contrast, minimal body weights and fat levels for female athletes have not been firmly established. Lohman (1992) suggests *fat values ranging from 12 %BF to 16 %BF for most female athletes, depending on the sport.* At levels less than 16 %BF, some women become amenorrheic (less than three menstrual periods per year), which may lead to bone mineral loss over extended periods of time. Although physical activity is positively associated with bone mineral content, amenorrheic athletes tend to have significantly less bone mineral content than eumenorrheic (10 to 13 menstrual periods per year) athletes and sedentary women (Drinkwater et al., 1984; Snow-Harter, 1993). Thus, the risk of stress fractures and premature osteoporosis is increased for amenorrheic athletes. However, more research is needed to fully understand the role of body fat and body weight in athletic amenorrhea.

The prevalence of amenorrhea is higher in the athletic population (3.4% to 66%) than in the general female population (2% to 5%) (Nattiv, Agostina, Drinkwater, & Yeager, 1993). Athletic amenorrhea is a complex, multifaceted phenomenon that is related not only to body fat and body weight, but to factors such as delayed menarche, eating disorders, nutrition, intensity and volume of training, and psychological stress (Sanborn, 1986; Yeager, Agostina, Nattiv, & Drinkwater, 1993).

Although there may be an optimal body weight and body composition to maximize performance in certain sports, athletes, coaches, athletic trainers, and exercise scientists need to recognize that these values may vary among individual athletes. Thus, *it is wiser to set individual goals for athletes that fall within a range of body fat values than to expect all athletes in a given sport to achieve the same level of body fatness.* Otherwise, some athletes may feel pressured to engage in unsafe weight-loss practices or may develop eating disorders in an attempt to meet unrealistic weight and fat loss goals. This pressure to excel and to maintain an "ideal" body weight and optimal level of body fat can place the athlete, particularly female athletes, at risk for the "female triad"—*eating disorders, amenorrhea, and premature osteoporosis.* When all three aspects of the triad are present, it may have a serious impact on the athlete's health and risk of mortality (Yeager et al., 1993).

We recommend that the athlete's body composition be assessed at the beginning and end of the off-season training period. Coaches are encouraged to seek the advice of team physicians, sport nutritionists, exercise physiologists, and athletic trainers for screening athletes for the "female triad" and in developing dietary recommendations for weight loss, weight gain, and exercise prescriptions for fat loss and fat-free mass (FFM) gains during the off-season.

In this chapter, body composition methods and prediction equations (Table 10.1) for physically active individuals and athletes are presented. These equations were selected based on the criteria outlined in chapter 1. Recommended equations are summarized in the Quick Reference Guide in Appendix A. To assess the body composition of male and female athletes, the skinfold, bioelectrical impedance, or anthropometric methods can be used.

Fat-Free Body Composition of Athletes

Physical activity and exercise training result in moderate weight loss, moderate-to-large losses in body fat, and small-to-moderate gains in fat-free mass

Table 10.1   Prediction Equations for Athletes

Method	Sport	Gender	Equation	Reference
SKF	All	Women (18-29 yr)	1. Db (g/cc)[a] = $1.096095 - 0.0006952\ (\Sigma 4SKF) + 0.0000011\ (\Sigma 4SKF)^2 - 0.0000714\ (age)$	Jackson et al. (1980)
	All	Boys (14-19 yr)	2. Db (g/cc)[a] = $1.10647 - 0.00162\ (subscapular\ SKF) - 0.00144\ (abdomen\ SKF) - 0.00077\ (triceps\ SKF) + 0.00071\ (midaxillary\ SKF)$	Forsyth & Sinning (1973)
	All	Men (18-29 yr)	3. Db (g/cc)[a] = $1.112 - 0.00043499\ (\Sigma 7SKF) + 0.00000055\ (\Sigma 7SKF)^2 - 0.00028826\ (age)$	Jackson & Pollock (1978)
BIA	All	Women (NR)	4. FFM (kg) = $0.73\ (HT^2/R) + 0.23\ (X_c) + 0.16\ (BW) + 2.0$	Houtkooper, Going, et al. (1989)
	All	Women (college)	5. FFM (kg) = $0.73\ (HT^2/R) + 0.116\ (BW) + 0.096\ (X_c) - 4.03$	Lukaski & Bolonchuk (1987)
	All	Men (college)	6. FFM (kg) = $0.734\ (HT^2/R) + 0.116\ (BW) + 0.096\ (X_c) - 3.152$	Lukaski & Bolonchuk (1987)
	All	Men (19-40 yr)	7. FFM (kg) = $1.949 + 0.701\ (BW) + 0.186\ (HT^2/R)$	Oppliger, Nielsen, Hoegh, et al. (1991)

(continued)

Table 10.1 (continued)

Method	Sport	Gender	Equation	Reference
Anthropometry	All	Women (18-23 yr)	8. FFM (kg) = 0.757 (BW) + 0.981 (neck C) − 0.516 (thigh C) + 0.79	Mayhew et al. (1983)
	Ballet	Girls and Women (11-25 yr)	9. FFM (kg) = 0.73 (BW) + 3.0	Hergenroeder et al. (1993)
	Wrestling	Boys (13-18 yr)	10. Db (g/cc)^a = 1.12691 − 0.00357 (arm C) − 0.00127 (AB C) + 0.00524 (forearm C)	Katch & McArdle (1973)
	Football	White men (18-23 yr)	11. %BF = 55.2 + 0.481 (BW) − 0.468 (HT)	Hortobagyi, Israel, Houmard, O'Brien, et al. (1992)

Σ4SKF (mm) = sum of four skinfolds: triceps + anterior suprailiac + abdomen + thigh; Σ7SKF (mm) = sum of seven skinfolds: chest + midaxillary + triceps + subscapular + abdomen + anterior suprailiac + thigh; HT = height (cm); R = resistance (Ω); X_c = reactance (Ω); BW = body weight (kg); C = circumference (cm); thigh C (cm) at the gluteal fold; AB C (cm): average abdominal circumference = [(AB$_1$ + AB$_2$)/2], where AB$_1$ (cm) = abdominal circumference anteriorly midway between the xyphoid process of the sternum and the umbilicus and laterally between the lower end of the rib cage and iliac crests, and AB$_2$ (cm) = abdominal circumference at the umbilicus level; NR = not reported

^{a}Use the following formulas to convert Db to %BF: Men %BF = [(4.95/Db) − 4.50] × 100, Women %BF = [(5.01/Db) − 4.57] × 100, Boys (7-12 yr) %BF = [(5.30/Db) − 4.89] × 100, Boys (13-16 yr) %BF = [(5.07/Db) − 4.64] × 100, Boys (17-19 yr) %BF = [(4.99/Db) − 4.55] × 100

(Wilmore, 1983). The degree of alteration in body composition depends on the mode of exercise, as well as the frequency, intensity, and duration of training. Cross-sectional studies indicate that physically active individuals and athletes have greater bone mineral content, bone density, and skeletal muscle mass (Aloia et al., 1978; Nilsson & Westlin, 1971). Thus, it is likely that the density of the FFB in athletic men and women will be greater than that of their sedentary counterparts.

However, the FFB density of physically active women with chronic, athletic amenorrhea may actually be less than sedentary women due to significant loss of bone mineral content (BMC) (Sanborn & Wagner, 1987). Bunt et al. (1990) reported that two-component model equations overestimated the relative body fatness (%BF) of amenorrheic runners with low BMC by as much as 3 %BF. On the other hand, the %BF of female bodybuilders with high BMC was underestimated by 3 %BF. They suggested using multicomponent model equations to account for interindividual variability in FFB composition in order to obtain more accurate estimations of body fatness in physically active, female populations. Unfortunately, almost all of the body composition prediction equations developed for athletes are based on two-component models, and there are limited data describing the composition and density of the FFB in physically active women and men.

Skinfold Equations for Athletes

Although there are sport-specific skinfold (SKF) equations to estimate body composition of athletes in certain sports (e.g., basketball, gymastics, and wrestling), research indicates that population-specific and generalized SKF equations developed for women and men accurately estimate the body density (Db) of athletes in many different sports (Hortobagyi, Israel, Houmard, O'Brien, et al., 1992; Oppliger, Nielsen, Shelter, Crowley, & Albright, 1992; Sinning et al., 1985; Sinning & Wilson, 1984; Thorland et al., 1991; Withers, Whittingham, et al., 1987).

The generalized sum of seven skinfolds (Σ7SKF) equation of Jackson and Pollock (1978) has been shown to accurately estimate the average body fatness of physically active men (Israel et al., 1989), black and white collegiate football players (Hortobagyi, Israel, Houmard, O'Brien, et al., 1992; Houmard et al., 1991), and males participating in 12 different collegiate sports (Sinning et al., 1985). The prediction error of this equation ranged from 2.2 %BF to 2.9 %BF. In comparison, the SKF equations of Katch and McArdle (1973) and Sloan (1967) accurately estimated average body fatness of elite, Australian athletes participating in 18 different sports (Withers, Craig, Bourdon, & Norton, 1987) and collegiate football players (Oppliger et al., 1992), but with slightly larger prediction errors (SEE = 2.9 %BF to 3.5 %BF). Clark, Kuta, Sullivan, Bedford, Penner, and Studesville (1993) reported that the Lohman

SKF equation, modified for wrestlers by Thorland et al. (1991), slightly overestimated the average minimal body weight of high school wrestlers by 0.6 kg; however, the prediction error was acceptable (SEE = 2.1 kg). For male adolescent athletes, 14 to 19 years of age, Thorland, Johnson, Tharp, Fagot, and Hammer (1984) recommended using the SKF equations of Forsyth and Sinning (1973), Lohman (1981), and Pollock, Schmidt, and Jackson (1980). For these equations, the standard deviation of the predicted Db from the Forsyth and Sinning equation more closely resembled that of the measured Db in their sample.

For female athletes, we recommend using the generalized Σ4SKF equation of Jackson, Pollock, and Ward (1980). Sinning and Wilson (1984) reported that this equation accurately estimated the average body fatness of female athletes participating in 10 different collegiate sports (SEE = 3.2 %BF). Likewise, Thorland et al. (1984) noted that this equation accurately predicted the average Db (SEE = 0.0072 g/cc) of female, adolescent athletes, ages 11 to 19 years. In comparison, the Σ7SKF and gluteal circumference equation, developed by Jackson et al. (1980), had a slightly higher prediction error (SEE = 3.7 %BF) in estimating the body fatness of elite, female athletes from Australia who competed in 14 different sports (Withers, Whittingham, et al., 1987). Of the 11 SKF equations cross-validated in their study, an equation developed for Japanese Native women (Nagamine & Suzuki, 1964; see chapter 8) yielded the smallest prediction error (SEE = 3.1 %BF).

In summary, *we recommend using the Jackson and Pollock Σ7SKF and the Forsyth and Sinning SKF equations, respectively, to estimate the body composition of adult and adolescent male athletes. For adult and adolescent female athletes, the Jackson et al. Σ4SKF equation should be used.* These equations are presented in Table 10.1 and in the Quick Reference Guide in Appendix A.

Bioelectrical Impedance Equations for Athletes

Many population-specific and generalized bioelectrical impedance (BIA) equations developed for the average population have been tested on athletic samples. Overall, cross-validation results indicate that these equations cannot be used to accurately estimate the fat-free mass (FFM) of athletic men and women. The equations of Deurenberg, Westrate, and van der Kooy (1989a); Deurenberg, van der Kooy, et al. (1991); Heitmann (1990); Kushner and Schoeller (1986); Lukaski et al. (1985, 1986); and Segal et al. (1988) systematically underestimated the FFM of black and white collegiate football players (Hortobagyi, Israel, Houmard, O'Brien, et al., 1992) and lean (3 %BF to 13 %BF), white men (Eckerson et al., 1992) by as much as 14 kg. Also, the prediction errors (SEEs) ranged from 2.9 to 6.3 kg. Likewise, BIA manufacturers' equations (BMR, RJL, and Valhalla) significantly underestimated the FFM of black and white football players (Oppliger et al., 1992) and male and female bodybuilders (Colville, Heyward, & Sandoval, 1989) by 3.8 to 4.8 kg, with SEEs ranging from 3.3 to 5.8 kg.

In contrast, Lukaski, Bolonchuk, Siders, and Hall (1990) reported that a BIA equation developed for women and men, 18 to 74 years of age (Lukaski & Bolonchuk, 1987), accurately predicted the average FFM of female and male collegiate athletes (SEE = 2.0 kg). Compared to most BIA equations for the general population, this equation had a higher regression coefficient for resistance index (0.734) and a lower one for body weight (0.116). Houtkooper, Going, et al. (1989) also reported similar coefficients (0.73 and 0.16, respectively, for resistance index and body weight) for an equation developed to estimate the FFM of lean and athletic women.

Eckerson et al. (1992) found that a BIA equation developed for high school wrestlers (Oppliger, Nielsen, Hoegh, & Vance, 1991) could be used to predict the FFM of lean men (SEE = 1.70 kg), ages 19 to 40 years. However, they reported that body weight alone accounted for 96% of the variance in FFM and had a slightly smaller prediction error (SEE = 1.68 kg) than the Oppliger equation. Similarly, Hergenroeder, Brown, and Klish (1993) noted that the average FFM of female ballet dancers, measured by the total body electrical conductivity method, was accurately estimated by body weight alone (SEE = 1.5 kg). The addition of bioimpedance measures did not improve the predictive accuracy of this equation. These findings suggest that FFM accounts for much of the total body weight in lean individuals, regardless of gender.

Based on these studies, *we recommend using the BIA equations of either Lukaski and Bolonchuk or Oppliger to estimate the FFM of lean, athletic men. For physically active women, we suggest the Houtkooper equation. For female ballet dancers,* FFM can be assessed using Hergenroeder's equation. These equations are presented in Table 10.1 and in the Quick Reference Guide.

Near-Infrared Interactance Equations for Athletes

Cross-validation of the Futrex-5000 manufacturer's near-infrared inter-actance (NIR) equation indicates that this equation systematically underestimates the body fatness of physically active men (Israel et al., 1989) and black and white collegiate football players (Hortobagyi et al., 1992b; Houmard et al., 1991), with prediction errors ranging from 3.6 %BF to 4.2 %BF. To our knowledge, no one has tested the predictive accuracy of this equation for athletic women.

Hortobagyi, Israel, Houmard, O'Brien, et al. (1992) developed separate NIR equations for black and white football players. For blacks, body weight and the optical density at the biceps site accounted for 87% of the variance in %BF, with an acceptable prediction error (SEE = 2.7 %BF). For white football players, optical density measures failed to improve the predictive accuracy of the equation beyond that explained by body weight and height only (SEE = 2.3 %BF). These equations need to be cross-validated on additional samples of football players before recommending their use.

Anthropometric Equations for Athletes

In general, the predictive accuracy of anthropometric equations is not as good as skinfold (SKF) equations for assessing the body composition of athletic women and men. Forsyth and Sinning (1973) reported large prediction errors when body density (Db) was estimated from combinations of skeletal breadth measures (SEE = 0.10 g/cc). However, Thorland et al. (1991) noted that the Db of high school wrestlers is accurately estimated using the anthropometric equations developed by Katch and McArdle (1973). On the other hand, Thorland et al. (1984) found that the Katch and McArdle equation does not adequately estimate the Db of adolescent male and female athletes. In addition, Mayhew, Piper, Koss, and Montaldi (1983) developed an anthropometric equation to predict fat-free mass (FFM) of female collegiate athletes participating in seven different sports. Using a combination of body weight, neck circumference, and thigh circumference as predictors, this equation accurately estimated average FFM (SEE = 2.6 kg), but, the size of their cross-validation sample (N = 32) was relatively small.

As mentioned previously, researchers have noted that the body composition of some athletes, such as ballet dancers and football players, is adequately estimated from body weight and stature only (Hergenroeder et al., 1993; Hortobagyi, Israel, Houmard, O'Brien, et al., 1992). Although anthropometric equations can be used to estimate body composition of high school wrestlers, female ballet dancers, and female athletes, there does not appear to be any anthropometric equations that are generalizable to the population of male athletes as a whole. *When SKFs cannot be measured, we suggest using the anthropometric equations presented in Table 10.1 to assess the body composition of athletes in certain sports.*

Prediction of Competitive and Minimal Body Weight

Once the body composition of the athlete is measured, you can use this information to determine the competitive or miminal body weight (MW) for the athlete. Minimal body weight is the body weight corresponding to 5 %BF for male and 12 %BF for females. Competitive body weight is based on the athlete's present fat-free mass (FFM) and desired %BF level. The athlete's %BF goal should fall within the range reported for athletes in a given sport (Table 10.2). In Figure 10.1, a sample calculation of competitive body weight for a female bodybuilder is illustrated. Assuming that her FFM

Table 10.2   Average Body Fat of Male and Female Athletes

Sport	Females %BF	Males %BF
Ballet dancing	13-20	8-14
Baseball		12-15
Basketball	20-27	7-11
Bodybuilding	9-13	6-9
Cycling	15	8-10
Football		
Backs		9-12
Linebackers		13-14
Linemen		16-19
Quarterbacks/kickers		14
Gymnastics	10-17	5-10
Ice hockey		8-15
Racquetball	14	8-9
Rock climbing	10-15	5-10
Skiing		
Alpine	21	7-14
Cross-country	16-22	7-12
Jumping		14
Soccer		10
Softball	22	
Speed skating	15-24	11
Swimming	14-24	9-12
Tennis	20	15-16
Track and field		
Discus throwers	25	16
Jumpers	8-14	7-8
Long distance runners	10-19	6-13
Middle distance runners	10-14	7-12
Shot putters	20-28	16-20
Sprinters	11-19	8-16
Decathletes		8-9
Pentathletes	11	
Volleyball	16-25	11-12
Weightlifting		
Power lifters		9-16
Olympic lifters		10-12
Wrestling		5-12
Rowing	14-18	8-15
Triathlon	7-17	5-11

Note. Data from Fleck (1983, pp. 399-400) and Wilmore (1983, pp. 23-24).

Athlete: female bodybuilder

Precompetition data   *Competition goals*
Body weight = 130 lb   Body weight = 123 lb
%BF = 15%   %BF = 10%
FFM = 110.5 lb   FFM = 110.5 lb

Steps:

1. Calculate the present FFM of the athlete: 130 lb × .85 = 110.5 lb
2. Set a reasonable competitive %BF goal for the athlete based on a value that falls within the range reported for female bodybuilders (see Table 10.2): 10% BF
3. Calculate the athlete's competitive body weight by dividing her present FFM by the competitive percent FFM (90% FFM): 110.5 lb/.90 = 123 lb
4. Calculate the athlete's body weight loss by subtracting the competitive body weight from the precompetitive body weight: 130 − 123 = 7 lb

---

Figure 10.1   Sample calculation of competitive body weight using the body composition method.

does not change, this athlete must lose 7 lb (fat and water weight) to achieve her competitive body weight and body fat goals.

In addition to using this approach to estimate competitive body weight, researchers have tested the applicability of skinfold (SKF), bioelectrical impedance (BIA), near-infrared interactance (NIR), and anthropometric methods for predicting minimal body weight (MW) of wrestlers. These equations were developed using two-component model estimates of FFM, and MW was based on a minimal fat level of 5 %BF for wrestlers (MW = FFM × 1.05). Research suggests that two-component model reference measures of FFM can be used to develop equations to predict MW of adolescent, male athletes. Horswill et al. (1990) reported that multicomponent models that adjust body density (Db) for hydration and mineral status did not improve estimates of MW in adolescent males compared to the two-component model. In judging the accuracy of these MW equations, the prediction error should not exceed 2.0 kg given that competitive weight-class intervals for high school wrestlers are 2.5 to 3.0 kg (Thorland, Johnson, Cisar, & Housh, 1987).

Oppliger, Nielsen, and Vance (1991) compared the predictive accuracy of anthropometric (Tcheng-Tipton and Oppliger-Tipton equations), SKF (Tipton-Oppliger equation), and BIA (BMR, RJL, and Valhalla manufacturers' equations) methods in estimating the MW of high school wrestlers. Using Thorland's (1987) criterion (SEE = ≤ 2.0 kg), only the Tipton and Oppliger (1984) SKF equation closely estimated the MW of their sample (SEE = 1.8 kg). Likewise, Clark, Kuta, Sullivan, et al. (1993) reported Lohman's sum of three skinfold (Σ3SKF) equation, which was modified for wrestlers by Thorland

Table 10.3   Prediction Equations for Estimation of Minimal Wrestling Weight

Method	Gender	Equation	Reference
SKF (*triceps + subscapular + abdomen*)	Male (high school & collegiate)	1. $Db (g/cc)^a = 1.0973 - 0.000815 (\sum 3SKF)$ $+ 0.00000084 (\sum 3SKF)^2$	Lohman[b] (1981)

	Male
	(high school
	& collegiate)
		2. $\%BF = 0.148$ (chest SKF) + 0.075 (subscapular SKF)
		     $+ 0.077$ (triceps SKF) + 0.160 (suprailiac SKF)
		     $+ 0.152$ (abdomen SKF) + 0.102 (thigh SKF)
			Tipton & Oppliger (1984)

$\sum 3SKF$ = sum of three skinfolds (mm)

[a]To convert Db to %BF, use the following equations: 13-16 yr $\%BF = [(5.07/Db) - 4.64] \times 100$, 17-19 yr $\%BF = [(4.99/Db) - 4.51] \times 100$, ≥ 20 yr $\%BF = [(4.95/Db) - 4.50] \times 100$

[b]Modified by Thorland et al. (1991) for high school wrestlers

(1991), could be used to predict MW for wrestlers (SEE = 2.1 kg). In contrast, BIA (RJL equation), NIR (Futrex-5000 equation), and dual-energy x-ray absorptiometry methods yielded large, unacceptable prediction errors (SEE = 2.6 to 3.5 kg) for their sample. Based on these studies, *we recommend using either the Tipton-Oppliger or modified Lohman SKF equations to assess the MW of high school wrestlers.* These equations are presented in Table 10.3 and in the Quick Reference Guide in Appendix A.

KEY POINTS

- The FFB density of physically active individuals and athletes is probably greater than that of sedentary individuals, given that athletes have relatively greater bone mineral content, bone density, and skeletal muscle mass.

- The generalized skinfold equations of Jackson et al. (Σ7SKF and Σ4SKF) can be used to assess the body composition of adult and adolescent male and female athletes.

- BIA equations developed specifically for physically active individuals yield more accurate estimations of body composition in athletes than equations developed for the general population.

- The NIR method should not be used to assess the body composition of physically active individuals or athletes.

- Body composition data can be used to predict competitive and mimimal body weight for athletes.

- The SKF method is preferable to BIA, NIR, and anthropometric methods for estimating the minimal body weight of wrestlers.

Chapter 11

Assessing Body Composition Changes

To set appropriate, individualized goals for clients in weight management and exercise training programs, it is important to have an accurate initial assessment of their body composition. In addition, changes in body composition due to weight loss or training need to be measured in order to modify weight goals of each client throughout weight reduction and exercise training programs and to evaluate the effectiveness of the weight loss or training regimen. However, assessing changes in body composition is problematic, especially when two-component models or prediction equations based on these models are used (Lohman, Going, & Houtkooper, 1988). In this chapter, the validity of using field methods to evaluate changes in the body composition of individuals participating in weight loss programs is addressed.

Total body density (Db) is affected not only by losses in fat mass, but by concomitant changes in muscle mass and total body water. Oftentimes, fat-free mass (FFM) decreases along with fat mass when severely obese clients consume a very low-calorie diet (Deurenberg, Westrate, & Hautvast, 1989; Kushner et al., 1990; van der Kooy et al., 1992; Vazquez & Janosky, 1991). The loss of FFM due to reductions in total body water (TBW) and muscle mass lowers fat-free body (FFB) and Db. Therefore, measures of Db will underestimate the fat loss of your client. This points to the importance of using multicomponent body composition models in order to accurately quantify changes in FFB composition during weight loss. Unfortunately, most of the research to date used reference methods and prediction equations based on two-component models. Thus, there is much debate as to whether or not field methods (skinfold, bioelectrical impedance, and anthropometry) can be used to monitor and predict changes in body composition during substantial weight loss (Deurenberg, Westrate, Hautvast, & van der Kooy, 1991; Deurenberg, Westrate, & van der Kooy, 1989a; Forbes, Simon, & Amatruda, 1992; Kushner et al., 1990; Mazess, 1991; Paijmans et al., 1992; Schoeller & Kushner, 1991; Vazquez & Janosky, 1991).

Skinfold Method

As mentioned earlier in this chapter, the skinfold (SKF) method is not recommended for assessing the body composition of obese clients primarily because of the difficulty in accurately measuring large SKFs. Also, the SKF method should not be used to assess body composition changes with weight loss for a number of reasons. First, this method assumes that the ratio of internal to subcutaneous fat is constant within and between individuals. However, in obese clients who undergo rapid and substantial weight loss, there may be a disproportionate decrease in internal fat compared to subcutaneous fat (Scherf, Franklin, Lucas, Stevenson, & Rubenfire, 1986). Secondly, relative decreases in SKF thickness during weight loss may not be the same at various sites (Ross, Leger, Marliss, Morris, & Gougeon, 1991). Thus, changes in SKF thickness are not highly correlated (r = 0.02 to 0.38) with weight loss (Bray et al., 1978).

Compared to two-component model reference measures, many SKF prediction equations underestimate the %BF of obese individuals before weight loss. Paijmans et al. (1992) reported that the average %BF of formerly obese individuals was significantly underestimated after weight loss using age-specific SKF equations (Sloan, 1967; Sloan, Burt, & Blyth, 1962) and generalized sum of three skinfold (Σ3SKF) equations (Jackson & Pollock, 1978; Jackson et al., 1980). These equations had large prediction errors (standard errors of estimate or SEE = 7.2 %BF to 10.2 %BF) as well. Although the SKF equations of Durnin and Womersley (1974) and Durnin and Rahaman (1967) accurately estimated average %BF, the prediction errors were not acceptable (SEE = 4.5 %BF to 5.0 %BF).

In addition, SKF equations do not adequately assess body composition changes during weight loss. Kushner et al. (1990) noted that the Jackson Σ7SKF equation significantly underestimated the change in FFM of obese women who consumed a very low calorie diet (520 kcal/day) or a hypocaloric diet (1000 to 1200 kcal/day). However, it is likely that their two-component reference method, total body water (TBW), overestimated the change in FFM given that the relative hydration of the FFM in obese clients is greater (76% FFM) than the value assumed for the two-component TBW equation (73% FFM). On the other hand, compared to hydrodensitometry, the Durnin and Womersley (1974) SKF equations significantly overestimated the loss of FFM in obese men and women on a low-calorie diet (van der Kooy et al., 1992). However, this SKF equation accurately estimated the average FFM of slightly obese men with an acceptable prediction error (SEE = 3.1 kg) both before and after a 10-week diet-exercise regimen (Ross et al., 1989). Compared to other studies, these subjects were not as severely obese and lost only 8 kg of body weight. The weight management program included a combination of exercise training and a moderately-restricted (1400 to 1800 kcal/day) diet for weight loss.

Bioelectrical Impedance Method

There is much debate over whether or not bioelectrical impedance (BIA) accurately predicts changes in fat-free mass (FFM) associated with weight loss. Although Ross et al. (1989) reported that the BIA equations of Lukaski (1987) and Segal et al. (1988) accurately estimated the average FFM of slightly obese men before and after weight loss, some researchers (Deurenberg, Westrate, & Hautvast, 1989; van der Kooy et al., 1992; Vazquez & Janosky, 1991) have noted that most BIA equations do not adequately reflect changes in FFM during weight loss compared to reference methods (hydrodensitometry and nitrogen balance). The BIA equations of Deurenberg et al. (1991), Gray et al. (1989), Kushner et al. (1990), Lukaski et al. (1986), and Segal et al. (1985, 1988) overestimated the change in FFM in obese men and women during weight loss (van der Kooy et al., 1992; Vazquez & Janosky, 1991). On the other hand, Deurenberg, Westrate, and Hautvast (1989) reported that their BIA equation significantly underestimated FFM loss in obese women compared to hydrodensitometry. They indicated, however, that part of this discrepancy between methods may be due to using the Siri two-component model to obtain reference measures of FFM in obese subjects. In contrast, Kushner et al. (1990) concluded that BIA may be a useful clinical method for measuring changes in body composition in obese women. In comparing estimates of FFM loss from measured total body water (TBW) and BIA equations, they noted that their BIA equation (Kushner & Schoeller, 1986) accurately predicted changes in FFM and TBW; the Deurenberg, Westrate, and van der Kooy (1989a) equation significantly understimated the average FFM loss.

Given these conflicting findings, *the validity of the BIA method for assessing changes in body composition remains questionable.* Forbes et al. (1992) reported that losses in FFM appear to be more highly related to changes in body weight (r = 0.69) than total body resistance (r = 0.56). In fact, resistance may increase, decrease, or stay the same during weight loss, depending on the ratio of change in FFM and body weight (ΔFFM/ΔBW). In the future, this issue may be resolved by using multicomponent body composition models to accurately quantify changes in FFB composition during weight loss. *Until this research is completed, we cannot recommend using the BIA method to monitor changes in the body composition of obese clients in weight management programs.*

Anthropometric Method

Although anthropometric equations accurately estimate the body composition of obese individuals (Weltman et al., 1987, 1988), there is little research documenting the use of these equations for assessing changes in body composition. However, compared to skinfolds, circumference measures are more highly related (r = 0.40 to 0.83) to weight loss (Bray et al., 1978).

Although individual circumferences reflect weight loss, the waist-to-hip ratio (WHR) does not change in response to rapid weight loss in individuals with upper-body obesity (WHR > 0.80 for women, WHR > 0.95 for men). Therefore, *WHR should not be used in clinical settings to assess changes in adipose tissue distribution during acute weight loss* (Ross et al., 1991). In addition, body mass index (BMI) does not adequately reflect changes in FFM during weight loss. Van der Kooy et al. (1992) reported that Deurenberg, Westrate, and Seidell's (1991) age- and gender-specific BMI equations significantly overestimated FFM loss in obese women and men consuming a hypocaloric diet.

In short, it appears that *SKF, BIA, and anthropometric (WHR and BMI) methods cannot be used to accurately estimate changes in body composition during weight loss.* However, in weight management programs, we recommend periodically measuring the circumferences of your clients and using somatograms (see chapter 5) to monitor changes in their anthropometric profiles.

KEY POINTS

- SKF equations do not accurately assess body composition changes during weight loss.
- BIA should not be used to monitor body composition changes of obese clients.
- Compared to SKFs, circumference measures are more highly associated with weight loss.
- SKFs and circumferences can be measured to monitor changes in your client's anthropometric profile.

Epilogue

In synthesizing and summarizing the research for this book, a number of voids in the research dealing with body composition assessment surfaced. In this section, we would like to identify these areas and highlight some future directions for body composition research.

First, use of multicomponent body composition models to quantify the components of the fat-free body and to develop prediction equations based on these models needs to be continued and refined. This will improve the predictive accuracy of practical body composition methods and equations used in clinical and field settings. Equations based on multicomponent models will enable us not only to accurately assess the body composition of healthy individuals but also to monitor changes in body composition during weight loss, pregnancy, and exercise training. In the future, we will be able to more precisely quantify alterations in the fat and fat-free body components resulting from spinal cord injuries and diseases such as AIDS, anorexia nervosa, cancer, cystic fibrosis, obesity, and renal failure. This will help health, fitness, and medical professionals in prescribing more effective nutrition, exercise, and medical interventions for treating these diseases.

Eventually, we will be able to accurately assess whole body composition *in vivo* using advanced technologies such as dual-energy x-ray absorptiometry (DXA) and multifrequency bioelectrical impedance analysis (BIA). The combination of these methods may ultimately replace, or at least refine, hydrodensitometry as the reference method. DXA provides measures of total body and regional bone mineral, bone density, and soft-tissue and lean-tissue masses. Multifrequency BIA has the potential for quantifying the volume of total body water and extracellular water. This will enable researchers and practitioners to detect relatively small changes in extracellular water and shifts in body water between the extracellular and intracellular fluid compartments. The information obtained from DXA and multifrequency bioelectrical impedance will further our understanding of how exercise, diet, and disease affect bone mineral and fluid distribution, as well as total body composition.

There is also a need to develop methods that are suitable for assessing regional body composition because of the strong link between intra-abdominal (visceral) fat and disease risk. DXA and segmental BIA methods appear to be good candidates for this purpose. The possibility of using practical anthropometric measures (circumferences and bony diameters) and anthropometric indexes, such as BMI, WHR, and the conicity index, to identify individuals at-risk because of upper-body obesity needs additional study.

With regard to practical assessment of body composition, we identified a number of prediction equations that need additional cross-validation to determine their applicability to certain population subgroups. These equations follow:

1. The BIA equations of Lohman (1992) and Gray et al. (1989) for elderly men and Baumgartner et al. (1991) for elderly women and men.
2. The SKF and NIR equations of Hicks, Heyward, Flores, et al. (1993) and the BIA equation of Stolarczyk et al. (1994) for American Indian women.
3. The SKF equations of Vickery et al. (1988) and Jackson and Pollock (1978) for black men.
4. The SKF equations of Jackson et al. (1978, 1980) for Hispanic women and men.
5. The BIA equations of Lohman (1992), Gray et al. (1989), Van Loan and Macylin (1987), and Segal et al. (1988) for Hispanic women and men.
6. The NIR equation of Heyward, Jenkins, et al. (1992) for white and Hispanic women.
7. The SKF and BIA equations of Wang et al. (1994, 1995) for Asian Americans.

In addition, there is a need to test the applicability of previously published skinfold, bioelectrical impedance, near-infrared interactance, and anthropometric prediction equations for assessing body composition of ethnic populations. If these equations are not generalizable to these groups, new equations should be developed using multicomponent models to obtain reference measures of body composition. Specifically, we have identified the following:

1. SKF equations for American Indian men, Hispanic and Asian American women and men, and anorexic women.
2. BIA equations for American Indian men and black, Hispanic, and Asian American men and women.
3. NIR equations for men, women, and children from all ethnic groups.
4. Anthropometric equations for the elderly, as well as American Indian, black, Hispanic, and Asian American men and women.

Quick Reference Guide

How to Use the Quick Reference Guide

This guide contains decision trees and equation finders to help you easily identify suitable body composition methods and equations for your clients. Use the decision trees to select methods and equations based on your client's (a) age, ethnicity, and gender (Figure A.1); (b) level of body fatness, ethnicity, and gender (Figure A.2); or (c) age, gender, and sport (Figure A.3). For example, if your client is a 35-year-old Hispanic male, use Figure A.1. Find your client's age in the "Age" row. Follow the arrows to the boxes corresponding to your client's ethnic group [**Hispanic**] and gender [**M = male**]. Continue following the arrow to boxes indicating suitable methods [**BIA**] and equations [**Go to Table 8.4, p. 121 or to p. 178**]. The BIA equation for this client can be found either in Table 8.4, p. 121 of text or on p. 178 of the Quick Reference Guide. To apply this equation, you will need to measure your client's height, body weight, age, and resistance.

If you are limited to one specific method for measuring body fat, you can find equations for that method by using the equation finders for the skinfold (Figure A.4a-b), bioelectrical impedance (Figure A.5a-b), near-infrared interactance (Figure A.6), and anthropometric (Figure A.7) methods. For example, if you are using the skinfold method to estimate the body fat of 48-year-old black women, go to the skinfold equation finder (Figure A.4b). In the section for adults, follow the arrows to the boxes corresponding the client's ethnicity [**Black**], gender and age [**Female, 18-55 yr**], and equation [**Jackson**]. The Jackson equation can be found either in Table 8.3 (see Equation 1 on p. 116 of text) or in the Quick Reference Guide on p. 177 (see Equation 1). To use this equation, you will need to know your client's age and the skinfold thicknesses at seven sites.

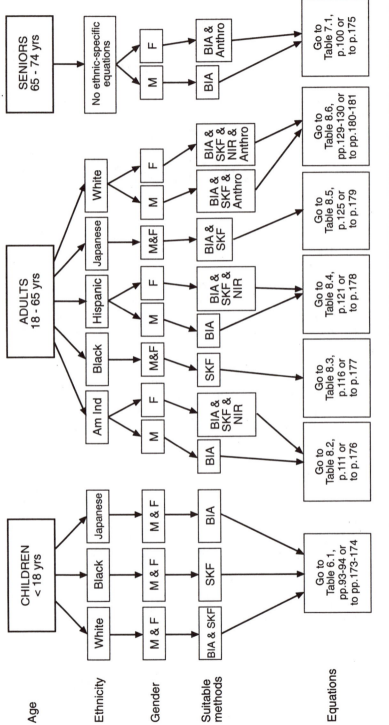

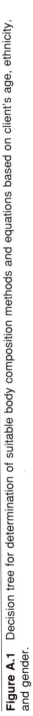

Figure A.1 Decision tree for determination of suitable body composition methods and equations based on client's age, ethnicity, and gender.

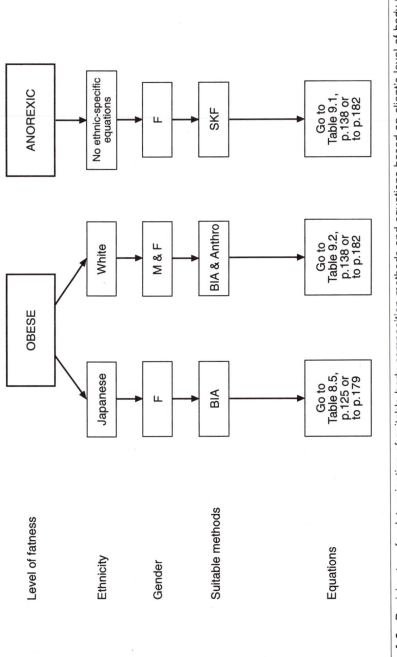

Figure A.2 Decision tree for determination of suitable body composition methods and equations based on client's level of fatness, ethnicity, and gender.

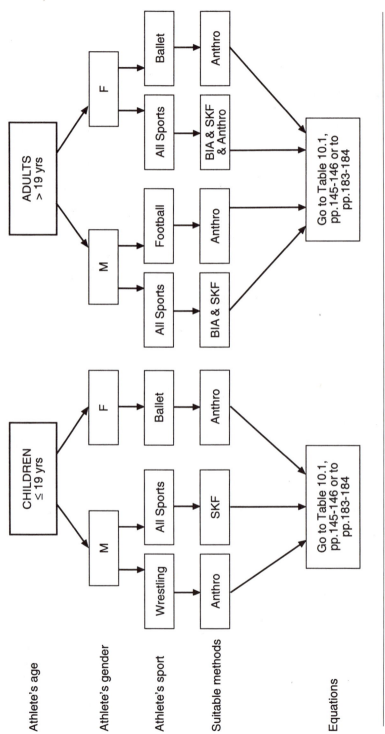

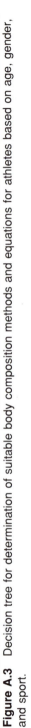

Figure A.3 Decision tree for determination of suitable body composition methods and equations for athletes based on age, gender, and sport.

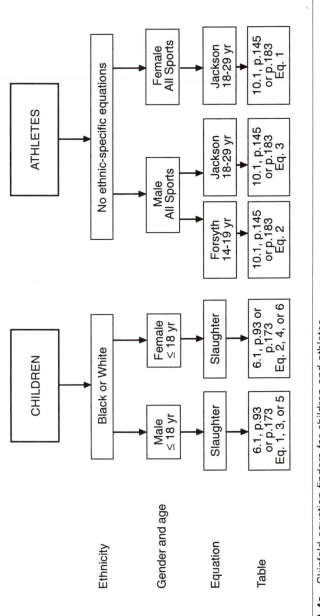

Figure A.4a   Skinfold equation finders for children and athletes.

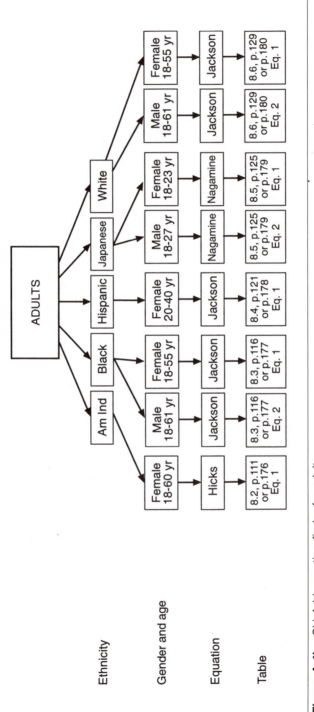

Figure A.4b   Skinfold equation finder for adults.

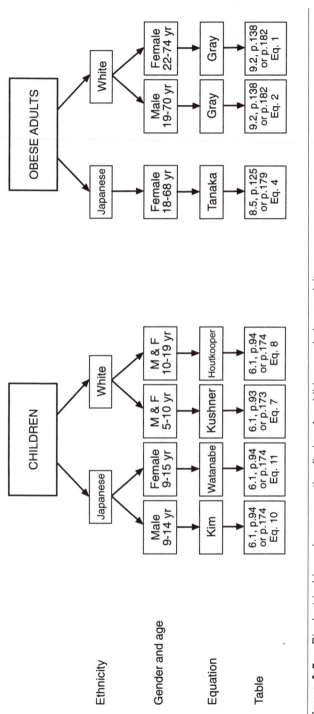

Figure A.5a Bioelectrical impedance equation finders for children and obese adults.

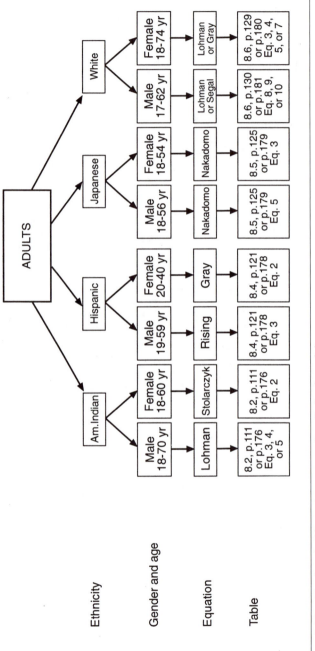

Figure A.5b   Bioelectrical impedance equation finder for adults.

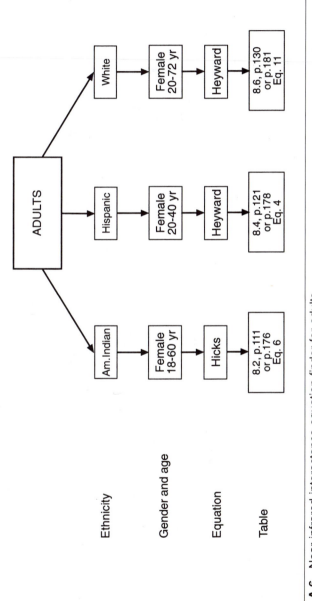

Figure A.6   Near-infrared interactance equation finder for adults.

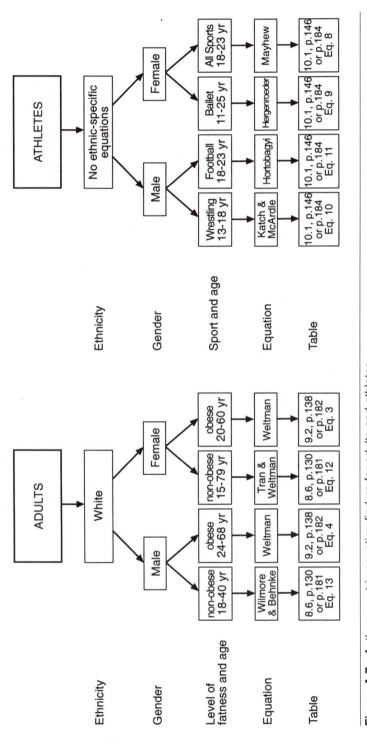

Figure A.7 Anthropometric equation finders for adults and athletes.

SYMBOL ABBREVIATIONS AND DEFINITIONS

	Symbol	Definition
GENERAL	%BF	Percent body fat
	BIA	Bioelectrical impedance analysis
	BMC (g)	Bone mineral content
	BMD (g/cm^2)	Bone mineral density
	BW (kg)	Body weight
	d (g/cc)	Density
	Db (g/cc)	Total body density
	DXA	Dual-energy x-ray absorptiometry
	FFB or FFM (kg)	Fat-free body or fat-free mass
	FIT index	Physical activity level
	FM (kg)	Fat mass
	HT (cm)	Height
	LBM (kg)	Lean body mass
	MW (kg)	Minimal body weight
	NIR	Near-infrared interactance
	SKF (mm)	Skinfold
	TBM (kg)	Total body mineral
	TBW (l)	Total body water
	$\dot{V}O_2max$	Maximum rate of oxygen consumption
SKF METHOD	ΣSKF (mm)	Sum of skinfolds
	Σ3SKF (mm)	Sum of three skinfolds
	Σ4SKF (mm)	Sum of four skinfolds
	Σ7SKF (mm)	Sum of seven skinfolds
BIA METHOD	HT^2/R	Resistance index
	p	Specific resistivity
	R (Ω)	Resistance
	X_c (Ω)	Reactance
	Z (Ω)	Impedance
NIR METHOD	OD	Optical density
	ΔOD_2	[OD$_2$ standard − OD$_2$ biceps]
ANTHROPOMETRY	AB C (cm)	Average abdominal circumference
	arm C (cm)	Arm circumference
	bi-iliac D (cm)	Bi-iliac diameter
	BMI (kg/m^2)	Body mass index
	C (cm)	Circumference
	C-index	Conicity index
	D (cm)	Bony diameter or bony width
	forearm C (cm)	Forearm circumference
	hip C (cm)	Hip circumference
	knee C (cm)	Knee circumference
	neck C (cm)	Neck circumference
	thigh C (cm)	Proximal thigh circumference
	WHR	Waist-to-hip ratio

MEASUREMENT	cc	Cubic centimeter
UNITS	cm	Centimeter
	g	Gram
	g/cc	Grams per cubic centimeter
	kcal	Kilocalorie
	kg	Kilogram
	kHz	Kilohertz
	l	Liter
	m	Meter
	MHz	Megahertz
	mm	Millimeter
	nm	Nanometer
	μA	Microampere
	$^{\circ}C$	Degree in Centigrade
	Ω	Ohm
	W	Watt
STATISTICAL	E	Total prediction error
TERMS	N	Sample size
	R_{mc}	Multiple correlation coefficient
	Σ	Sum of scores
	SEE	Standard error of estimate
	r	Correlation coefficient
	$r_{y,y'}$	Validity coefficient

Appendix A—Table 6.1   Prediction Equations for Children

Method	Ethnicity/gender	Equation	Reference
SKF			
$\Sigma triceps + calf$	Black and White		
	Boys (all ages)	1. $\%BF = 0.735\ (\Sigma SKF) + 1.0$	Slaughter et al. (1988)
	Girls (all ages)	2. $\%BF = 0.610\ (\Sigma SKF) + 5.1$	Slaughter et al. (1988)
$\Sigma triceps + subscapular$	Black and White		
$(\Sigma SKF > 35mm)$	Boys (all ages)	3. $\%BF = 0.783\ (\Sigma SKF) + 1.6$	Slaughter et al. (1988) ✗
	Girls (all ages)	4. $\%BF = 0.546\ (\Sigma SKF) + 9.7$	Slaughter et al. (1988)
$(\Sigma SKF < 35mm)$	Black and White		
	Boys (all ages)	5. $\%BF = 1.21\ (\Sigma SKF) - 0.008\ (\Sigma SKF)^2 + I^*$	Slaughter et al. (1988) ✗
	Girls (all ages)	6. $\%BF = 1.33\ (\Sigma SKF) - 0.013\ (\Sigma SKF)^2 - 2.5$	Slaughter et al. (1988)
BIA	White		
	Boys and girls (6-10 yr)	7. $TBW\ (l)^a = 0.593\ (HT^2/R) + 0.065\ (BW) + 0.04$	Kushner (1992)

(continued)

Appendix A—Table 6.1 (*continued*)

Method	Ethnicity/gender	Equation	Reference
BIA (*continued*)			
	White		
	Boys and girls (10-19 yr)	8. FFM (kg) = 0.61 (HT²/R) + 0.25 (BW) + 1.31	Houtkooper et al. (1992)
	Boys and girls (8-15 yr)	9. FFM (kg) = 0.62 (HT²/R) + 0.21 (BW) + 0.10 (X_c) + 4.2	Lohman (1992)
	Japanese Native		
	Boys (9-14 yr)	10. FFM (kg) = 0.56 (HT²/Z) + 0.20 (BW) + 1.66	Kim et al. (1993)
	Girls (9-15 yr)	11. FFM (kg) = 0.42 (HT²/Z) + 0.60 (BW) − 0.75 (arm C) + 7.72	Watanabe et al. (1993)

$\sum$SKF = sum of skinfolds (mm), HT = height (cm), BW = body weight (kg), R = resistance (Ω), X_c = reactance (Ω), Z = impedance (Ω), arm C = arm circumference (cm), TBW = total body water (l)

*I = intercept substitutions based on maturation and ethnicity for boys:

Age	Black	White
Prepubescent	−3.2	−1.7
Pubescent	−5.2	−3.4
Postpubescent	−6.8	−5.5

[a]To convert TBW to FFM, use the following age-gender hydration constants:

Boys: 5-6 yr FFM (kg) = TBW/0.77   Girls: 5-6 yr FFM (kg) = TBW/0.78
      7-8 yr FFM (kg) = TBW/0.768   7-8 yr FFM (kg) = TBW/0.776
      9-10 yr FFM (kg) = TBW/0.762   9-10 yr FFM (kg) = TBW/0.77

Appendix A—Table 7.1   Prediction Equations for Elderly

Method	Gender	Equation	Reference
BIA	Women		
	(50-70 yr)	1. FFM (kg) = 0.474 (HT^2/R) + 0.180 (BW) + 7.3	Lohman (1992)
	(22-74 yr)	2. FFM (kg) = 0.00151 (HT^2) – 0.0344 (R) + 0.140 (BW) – 0.158 (age) + 20.387	Gray et al. (1989)
	Men		
	(50-70 yr)	3. FFM (kg) = 0.600 (HT^2/R) + 0.186 (BW) + 0.226 (X_c) – 10.9	Lohman (1992)
	(19-70 yr)	4. FFM (kg) = 0.00139 (HT^2) – 0.0801 (R) + 0.187 (BW) + 39.83	Gray et al. (1989)
	Women		
	(65-94 yr)	5. FFM (kg) = 0.28 (HT^2/R) + 0.27 (BW) + 0.31 (thigh C) – 1.732	Baumgartner et al. (1991)
	Men		
	(65-94 yr)	6. FFM (kg) = 0.28 (HT^2/R) + 0.27 (BW) + 0.31 (thigh C) + 2.768	Baumgartner et al. (1991)
Anthropometry	Women		
	(15-79 yr)	7. Db (g/cc)[a] = 1.168297 – [0.002824 × AB C] + [0.0000122098 × (AB C)²] – [0.000733128 × hip C] + [0.000510477 × HT] – [0.000216161 × age]	Tran & Weltman (1989)

HT = height (cm); BW = body weight (kg); R = resistance (Ω); X_c = reactance (Ω); C = circumference (cm); AB C (cm): average abdominal circumference = [(AB$_1$ + AB$_2$)/2], where AB$_1$ (cm) = abdominal circumference anteriorly midway between the xiphoid process of the sternum and the umbilicus and laterally between the lower end of the rib cage and iliac crests, and AB$_2$ (cm) = abdominal circumference at the umbilicus level

[a]Use the following formula to convert Db to %BF: %BF = [(5.01/Db) – 4.57] × 100

Appendix A—Table 8.2   Prediction Equations for American Indians

Method	Gender	Equation	Reference
SKF (*triceps + midaxillary + suprailiac*)	Women (18-60 yr)	1. Db (g/cc)^a = 1.061983 − 0.000385 ($\sum$SKF) − 0.000204 (age)	Hicks, Heyward, Flores, et al. (1993)
BIA	Women (18-60 yr)	2. FFM (kg) = 0.1555 (BW) + 0.001254 (HT^2) − 0.04904 (R) + 0.1417 (X$_c$) − 0.0833 (age) + 20.05	Stolarczyk et al. (1994)
	Men (18-29 yr)	3. FFM (kg) = 0.485 (HT^2/R) + 0.338 (BW) + 5.32	Lohman (1992)
	(30-49 yr)	4. FFM (kg) = 0.549 (HT^2/R) + 0.163 (BW) + 0.092 (X$_c$) + 4.51	Lohman (1992)
	(50-70 yr)	5. FFM (kg) = 0.60 (HT^2/R) + 0.186 (BW) + 0.226 (X$_c$) − 10.9	Lohman (1992)
NIR (*pectoral + biceps*)	Women (18-60 yr)	6. Db (g/cc)^a = 1.070761 − 0.000987 (hip C) − 0.036986 ($\sum\Delta$OD$_2$) + 0.000417 (HT) + 0.000087 (FIT index) − 0.000189 (age)	Hicks, Heyward, Flores, et al. (1993)

$\sum$SKF = sum of skinfold (mm), BW = body weight (kg), HT = height (cm), R = resistance (Ω), X$_c$ = reactance (Ω), hip C = hip circumference (cm), $\sum\Delta$OD$_2$ = [(OD$_2$ standard − OD$_2$ pectoral) + (OD$_2$ standard − OD$_2$ biceps)], FIT index = physical activity level (see Figure 8.1, page 112)

^{a}Use the following formula to convert Db to %BF: %BF = [(4.81/Db) − 4.34] × 100

Appendix A—Table 8.3   Prediction Equations for Blacks

Method	Gender		Equation	Reference
SKF (*chest + abdomen + thigh* *+ triceps + subscapular +* *suprailiac + midaxillary*)	Women (18-55 yr)	1.	$Db \ (g/cc)^a = 1.0970 - 0.00046971 \ (\Sigma 7SKF) + 0.00000056 \ (\Sigma 7SKF)^2$ $\quad - 0.00012828 \ (age)$	Jackson et al. (1980)
	Men (18-61 yr)	2.	$Db \ (g/cc)^a = 1.1120 - 0.00043499 \ (\Sigma 7SKF) + 0.00000055 \ (\Sigma 7SKF)^2$ $\quad - 0.0002826 \ (age)$	Jackson & Pollock (1978)

$\Sigma 7SKF$ = sum of seven skinfolds (mm)

[a]Use the following formulas to convert Db to %BF: Men %BF = $[(4.37/Db) - 3.93] \times 100$, Women %BF = $[(4.85/Db) - 4.39] \times 100$

Appendix A—Table 8.4 Prediction Equations for Hispanics

Method	Gender	Equation	Reference
SKF (chest + abdomen + thigh + triceps + subscapular + suprailiac + midaxillary)	Women (20-40 yr)	1. Db (g/cc)[a] = $1.0970 - 0.00046971\ (\Sigma 7\text{SKF}) + 0.00000056\ (\Sigma 7\text{SKF})^2 - 0.00012828\ (\text{age})$	Jackson et al. (1980)
BIA	Women (20-40 yr)	2. FFM (kg) = $0.00151\ (\text{HT}^2) - 0.0344\ (\text{R}) + 0.140\ (\text{BW}) - 0.158\ (\text{age}) + 20.387$	Gray et al. (1989)
	Men (19-59 yr)	3. FFM (kg) = $13.74 + 0.34\ (\text{HT}^2/\text{R}) + 0.33\ (\text{BW}) - 0.14\ (\text{age}) + 6.18$	Rising et al. (1991)
NIR (biceps)	Women (20-40 yr)	4. Db (g/cc)[a] = $1.02823066 - 0.080035\ (\Delta\text{OD}_2) - 0.000459\ (\text{age}) - 0.000754\ (\text{BW}) + 0.000493\ (\text{HT})$	Heyward, Jenkins, et al. (1992)

$\Sigma 7$SKF = sum of seven skinfolds (mm), HT = height (cm), R = resistance (Ω), BW = body weight (kg), $\Delta\text{OD}_2 = (\text{OD}_2\ \text{standard} - \text{OD}_2\ \text{biceps})$, [a]Use the following formula to convert Db to %BF: %BF = $[(4.87/\text{Db}) - 4.41] \times 100$

Table 8.5 Prediction Equations for Japanese Natives

Method	Gender	Equation	Reference
SKF (*triceps + subscapular*)	Women (18-23 yr)	1. $Db (g/cc)^a = 1.0897 - 0.00133 (\sum SKF)$	Nagamine & Suzuki (1964)
	Men (18-27 yr)	2. $Db (g/cc)^a = 1.0913 - 0.00116 (\sum SKF)$	Nagamine & Suzuki (1964)
BIA	Women (18-54 yr)	3. $Db (g/cc)^a = 1.1628 - 0.1067 (BW \times Z/HT^2)$	Nakadomo et al. (1990)
	Obese women (18-68 yr) and (25-60 %BF)	4. $Db (g/cc)^a = 1.1307 - 0.0719 (BW \times Z/HT^2)$ $- 0.0003$ (age)	Tanaka et al. (1992)
	Men (18-56 yr)	5. $Db (g/cc)^a = 1.1492 - 0.0918 (BW \times Z/HT^2)$	Nakadomo et al. (1990)

$\sum SKF$ = sum of skinfolds (mm), BW = body weight (kg), Z = impedance (Ω), HT = height (cm)

[a]Use the following formulas to convert Db to %BF: Men (18-48 yr) %BF = $[(4.97/Db) - 4.52] \times 100$; Women (18-48 yr) %BF = $[(4.76/Db) - 4.28] \times 100$; Men (61-78 yr) %BF = $[(4.87/Db) - 4.41] \times 100$; Women (61-78 yr) %BF = $[(4.95/Db) - 4.50] \times 100$

Appendix A—Table 8.6 Prediction Equations for Whites

Method	Gender	Equation	Reference
SKF (*triceps + suprailiac + thigh*)	Women (18-55 yr)	1. $Db (g/cc)^a$ = 1.0994921 − 0.0009929 ($\sum 3SKF$) + 0.0000023 ($\sum 3SKF$)^2 − 0.0001392 (age)	Jackson et al. (1980)
(*chest + abdomen + thigh*)	Men (18-61 yr)	2. $Db (g/cc)^a$ = 1.109380 − 0.0008267 ($\sum 3SKF$) + 0.0000016 ($\sum 3SKF$)^2 − 0.0002574 (age)	Jackson & Pollock (1978)
BIA	Women		
	(18-29 yr)	3. FFM (kg) = 0.476 (HT^2/R) + 0.295 (BW) + 5.49	Lohman (1992)
	(30-49 yr)	4. FFM (kg) = 0.493 (HT^2/R) + 0.141 (BW) + 11.59	Lohman (1992)
	(50-70 yr)	5. FFM (kg) = 0.474 (HT^2/R) + 0.180 (BW) + 7.3	Lohman (1992)
	(18-64 yr)	6. FFM (kg) = 0.00085 (HT^2) − 0.02375 (R) + 0.3736 (BW) − 0.1531 (age) + 13.4947	Van Loan & Mayclin (1987)
	(22-74 yr)	7. FFM (kg) = 0.00151 (HT^2) − 0.0344 (R) + 0.140 (BW) − 0.158 (age) + 20.387	Gray et al. (1989)

Men		
(18-29 yr) (<20 %BF)	8. FFM (kg) = 0.485 (HT^2/R) + 0.338 (BW) + 5.32	Lohman (1992)
(17-62 yr) (≥20 %BF)	9. FFM (kg) = 0.00066360 (HT^2) − 0.02117 (R) + 0.62854 (BW) − 0.12380 (age) + 9.33285	Segal et al. (1988)
(17-62 yr)	10. FFM (kg) = 0.00088580 (HT^2) − 0.02999 (R) + 0.42688 (BW) − 0.07002 (age) + 14.52435	Segal et al. (1988)
NIR		
(biceps)		
Women		
(20-72 yr)	11. Db (g/cc)^a = 1.02823066 − 0.080035 (ΔOD$_2$) − 0.000459 (age) − 0.000754 (BW) + 0.000493 (HT)	Heyward, Jenkins et al. (1992)
Anthropometry		
Women		
(15-79 yr)	12. Db (g/cc)^a = 1.168297 − 0.002824 (AB C) + 0.0000122098 (AB C)^2 − 0.000733128 (hip C) + 0.000510477 (HT) − 0.000216161 (age)	Tran & Weltman (1989)
Men		
(18-40 yr)	13. FFM (kg) = 39.652 + 1.0932 (BW) + 0.8370 (bi-iliac D) + 0.3297 (AB$_1$ C) − 1.0008 (AB$_2$ C) − 0.6478 (knee C)	Wilmore & Behnke (1969)

Σ3SKF = sum of three skinfolds (mm); HT = height (cm); R = resistance (Ω); BW = body weight (kg); ΔOD$_2$ = (OD$_2$ standard − OD$_2$ biceps); C = circumference (cm), AB C (cm): average abdominal circumference = [(AB$_1$ + AB$_2$)/2], where AB$_1$ (cm) = abdominal circumference anteriorly midway between the xiphoid process of sternum and the umbilicus and laterally between the lower end of the rib cage and iliac crests, and AB$_2$ (cm) = abdominal circumference at the umbilicus level; D = diameter (cm)

[a]Use the following formulas to convert Db to %BF: Men %BF = [(4.95/Db) − 4.50] × 100, Women %BF = [(5.01/Db) − 4.57] × 100

Appendix A—Table 9.1   Prediction Equation for Anorexic Women

Method	Gender	Equation	Reference
SKF (*triceps + suprailiac + thigh*)	Women (18-55 yr)	1. Db (g/cc)[a] = 1.0994921 − 0.0009929 ($\sum$3SKF) + 0.0000023 ($\sum$3SKF)^2 − 0.0001392 (age)	Jackson et al. (1980)

$\sum$3SKF = sum of three skinfolds (mm)

[a]Use the following formula to convert Db to %BF: %BF = [(5.26/Db) − 4.83] × 100

Appendix A—Table 9.2   Prediction Equations for Obese Individuals

Method	Gender	Equation	Reference
BIA	Women (19-59 %BF)	1. FFM (kg) = 0.00151 (HT^2) − 0.0344 (R) + 0.140 (BW) − 0.158 (age) + 20.387	Gray et al. (1989)
	Men (9-45 %BF)	2. FFM (kg) = 0.00139 (HT^2) − 0.0801 (R) + 0.187 (BW) + 39.830	Gray et al. (1989)
Anthropometry	Women (20-60 yr)	3. %BF = 0.11077 (AB C) − 0.17666 (HT) + 0.14354 (BW) + 51.03301	Weltman et al. (1988)
	Men (24-68 yr)	4. %BF = 0.31457 (AB C) − 0.10969 (BW) + 10.8336	Weltman et al. (1987)

HT = height (cm); R = resistance (Ω); BW = body weight (kg); AB C (cm): average abdominal circumference = [(AB$_1$ + AB$_2$)/2], where AB$_1$ (cm) = abdominal circumference anteriorly midway between the xyphoid process of the sternum and the umbilicus and laterally between the lower end of the rib cage and iliac crests, and AB$_2$ (cm) = abdominal circumference at the umbilicus level

Appendix A—Table 10.1   Prediction Equations for Athletes

Method	Sport	Gender	Equation	Reference
SKF	All	Women (18-29 yr)	1. Db $(g/cc)^a$ = 1.096095 − 0.0006952 ($\sum$4SKF) + 0.0000011 $(\sum 4SKF)^2$ − 0.0000714 (age)	Jackson et al. (1980)
	All	Boys (14-19 yr)	2. Db $(g/cc)^a$ = 1.10647 − 0.00162 (subscapular SKF) − 0.00144 (abdomen SKF) − 0.00077 (triceps SKF) + 0.00071 (midaxillary SKF)	Forsyth & Sinning (1973)
	All	Men (18-29 yr)	3. Db $(g/cc)^a$ = 1.112 − 0.00043499 ($\sum$7SKF) + 0.00000055 $(\sum 7SKF)^2$ − 0.00028826 (age)	Jackson & Pollock (1978)
BIA	All	Women (NR)	4. FFM (kg) = 0.73 (HT^2/R) + 0.23 (X_c) + 0.16 (BW) + 2.0	Houtkooper, Going, et al. (1989)
	All	Women (college)	5. FFM (kg) = 0.73 (HT^2/R) + 0.116 (BW) + 0.096 (X_c) − 4.03	Lukaski & Bolonchuk (1987)
	All	Men (college)	6. FFM (kg) = 0.734 (HT^2/R) + 0.116 (BW) + 0.096 (X_c) − 3.152	Lukaski & Bolonchuk (1987)
	All	Men (19-40 yr)	7. FFM (kg) = 1.949 + 0.701 (BW) + 0.186 (HT^2/R)	Oppliger, Nielsen, Hoegh, et al. (1991)

(continued)

Appendix A—Prediction Equations

Appendix A—Table 10.1 (*continued*)

Method	Sport	Gender	Equation	Reference
Anthropometry	All	Women (18-23 yr)	8. FFM (kg) = 0.757 (BW) + 0.981 (neck C) – 0.516 (thigh C) + 0.79	Mayhew et al. (1983)
	Ballet	Girls and Women (11-25 yr)	9. FFM (kg) = 0.73 (BW) + 3.0	Hergenroeder et al. (1993)
	Wrestling	Boys (13-18 yr)	10. Db (g/cc)^a = 1.12691 – 0.00357 (arm C) – 0.00127 (AB C) + 0.00524 (forearm C)	Katch & McArdle (1973)
	Football	White men (18-23 yr)	11. %BF = 55.2 + 0.481 (BW) – 0.468 (HT)	Hortobagyi, Israel, Houmard, O'Brien, et al. (1992)

Σ4SKF (mm) = sum of four skinfolds: triceps + anterior suprailiac + abdomen + thigh; Σ7SKF (mm) = sum of seven skinfolds: chest + midaxillary + triceps + subscapular + abdomen + anterior suprailiac + thigh; HT = height (cm); R = resistance (Ω); X_c = reactance (Ω); BW = body weight (kg); C = circumference (cm); thigh C (cm) at the gluteal fold; AB C (cm): average abdominal circumference = [(AB$_1$ + AB$_2$)/2], where AB$_1$ (cm): abdominal circumference anteriorly midway between the xyphoid process of the sternum and the umbilicus and laterally between the lower end of the rib cage and iliac crests, and AB$_2$ (cm) = abdominal circumference at the umbilicus level; NR = not reported

^{a}Use the following formulas to convert Db to %BF: Men %BF = [(4.95/Db) – 4.50] × 100, Women %BF = [(5.01/Db) – 4.57] × 100, Boys (7-12 yr) %BF = [(5.30/Db) – 4.89] × 100, Boys (13-16 yr) %BF = [(5.07/Db) – 4.64] × 100, Boys (17-19 yr) %BF = [(4.99/Db) – 4.55] × 100

Appendix A—Table 10.3   Prediction Equations for Estimation of Minimal Wrestling Weight

Method	Gender	Equation	Reference
SKF (*triceps + subscapular + abdomen*)	Male (high school & collegiate)	1. Db (g/cc)[a] = 1.0973 − 0.000815 (Σ3SKF) + 0.00000084 (Σ3SKF)^2	Lohman[b] (1981)
	Male (high school & collegiate)	2. %BF = 0.148 (chest SKF) + 0.075 (subscapular SKF) + 0.077 (triceps SKF) + 0.160 (suprailiac SKF) + 0.152 (abdomen SKF) + 0.102 (thigh SKF)	Tipton & Oppliger (1984)

Σ3SKF = sum of three skinfolds (mm)

[a]To convert Db to %BF, use the following equations: 13-16 yr %BF = [(5.07/Db) − 4.64] × 100, 17-19 yr %BF = [(4.99/Db) − 4.55] × 100, ≥20 yr %BF = [(4.95/Db) − 4.50] × 100

[b]Modified by Thorland et al. (1991) for high school wrestlers

Sources for Body Composition Equipment

EQUIPMENT	SUPPLIERS
Anthropometers	
Spreading calipers Sliding calipers Standard skeletal anthropometer	Pfister Import-Export, Inc. 450 Barell Ave. Carlstadt, NJ 07072 Phone: (202) 939-4606
Anthropometric tape measure	Country Technology, Inc. P.O. Box 87 Gays Mills, WI 54631 Phone: (608) 735-4718
Bioimpedance analyzers RJL	RJL Systems 9930 Whittier Detroit, MI 48224 Phone: (800) 528-4513

Tri-Frequency

Daninger Medical Technology
4140 Fisher Rd.
Columbus, OH 43228
Phone: (614) 276-8267

Valhalla

Valhalla Scientific, Inc.
9955 Mesa Rim Rd.
San Diego, CA 92126
Phone: (800) 395-4565

Xitron-4000

Xitron Technologies
10225 Barnes Canyon Rd.,
Ste. A102
San Diego, CA 92121
Phone: (619) 458-9852

**Calibration instruments/
supplies**
Skinfold calibration blocks
  (15 mm)

Creative Health Products
5148 Saddle Ridge Rd.
Plymouth, MI 48170
Phone: (800) 742-4478

Standard calibration
  weights

Toledo Scale
431 Ohio Pike
Way Cross Office Park, Ste. 302
Toledo, OH
Phone: (513) 528-2300

Vernier caliper

L.S. Starrett Co.
121 Crescent St.
Athol, MA 01331
Phone: (508) 249-3551

**Dual-energy x-ray absorp-
tiometers**
Hologic QDR-1000

Hologic
590 Lincoln St.
Waltham, MA 02154
Phone: (800) 321-4654

Norland XR-26

Norland
W6340 Hackbarth Rd.
Fort Atkinson, WI 53538
Phone: (800) 333-8456

Lunar DPX

Lunar Radiation Corp.
313 W. Beltline Hwy.
Madison, WI 53713
Phone: (608) 274-2663

**Near-infrared interactance
analyzer**
Futrex

Futrex, Inc.
P.O. Box 2398
Gaithersburg, MD 20886
Phone: (800) 255-4206

Scales
Chatillon underwater
   weighing scale
Detecto balance beam scale
Health-O-Meter balance
   beam scale
Health-O-Meter digital scale
Seca digital scale

Creative Health Products
5148 Saddle Ridge Rd.
Plymouth, MI 48170
Phone: (800) 742-4478

Skinfold calipers
Adipometer (plastic)

Ross Laboratories
625 Cleveland Ave.
Columbus, OH 43216
Phone: (800) 344-9739

Fat-Control (plastic)

Creative Health Products
5148 Saddle Ridge Rd.
Plymouth, MI 48170
Phone: (800) 742-4478

Fat-O-Meter (plastic)

Health and Education Services
2442 Irving Park Rd.
Chicago, IL 60618
Phone: (312) 628-1787

Harpenden

Quinton Instruments
2121 Terry Ave.
Seattle, WA 98121
Phone: (800) 426-0538

Holtain

Pfister Import-Export, Inc.
450 Barell Ave.
Carlstadt, NJ 07072
Phone: (201) 939-4606

Lafayette	Creative Health Products 5148 Saddle Ridge Rd. Plymouth, MI 48170 Phone: (800) 742-4478
Lange	Cambridge Scientific Industries 527 Poplar St. Cambridge, MD 21613 Phone: (800) 638-9566
McGaw (plastic)	McGaw Laboratories, Inc. 2525 McGaw Ave. Irvine, CA 92714 Phone: (714) 660-2000
Slim-Guide (plastic)	Creative Health Products 5148 Saddle Ridge Rd. Plymouth, MI 48170 Phone: (800) 742-4478
Skyndex	Cramer Products P.O. Box 1001 Gardner, KS 66030 Phone: (913) 884-7511

Stadiometers

Harpenden stadiometer Holtain stadiometer	Pfister Import-Export, Inc. 450 Barell Ave. Carlstadt, NJ 07072 Phone: (201) 939-4606

Glossary

abdominal fat — Subcutaneous and visceral fat in the abdominal region of the body.

adipose tissue — Fat (~83%) plus its supporting structures (~2% protein and ~15% water).

amenorrhea — An abnormal menstrual cycle with three or less menstrual periods per year.

android obesity — Upper-body or abdominal obesity; pear-shaped; accumulation of adipose tissue on the trunk and abdomen.

anorexia nervosa — Disorder associated with abnormal eating patterns including food restriction, prolonged fasting, and use of diet pills, diuretics, and laxatives.

anthropometer — An instrument used to measure the breadth and length of body segments (e.g., standard anthropometer, small sliding caliper, and spreading caliper).

anthropometry — The measurement of body size and proportions, including skinfold thicknesses, circumferences, bony widths and lengths, stature, and body weight.

athletic amenorrhea — Exercise-induced cessation of menstrual periods (three or less periods per year).

bioelectrical impedance analysis (BIA) — A body composition method used to estimate total body water or fat-free mass by measuring the conductance of low-level electrical current through the body.

body density (Db) — The overall density of the fat, water, mineral, and protein components of the human body; total body mass expressed relative to total body volume.

body mass index (BMI) — A crude index of obesity; the ratio of body weight-to-height squared.

cadaver analysis — A method used to determine the water, mineral, lipid, and protein content of the human body.

calibration block — A block with a fixed, known width (e.g., 10, 15, and 20 mm) used to check the measurement accuracy of skinfold calipers and small sliding calipers.

capacitance — The storage of voltage for a brief moment in time.

conductance — The amount of electrical current that can be conducted by the body; dependent on the number of ions per unit volume.

conicity index (C-index) — A measure of the degree of deviation of the body's geometry from a perfect cylinder shape.

cross-validation — A statistical technique used to assess the validity of body composition methods and the predictive accuracy of body composition prediction equations.

dual-energy x-ray absorptiometry (DXA) — A body composition method used in clinical and research settings to estimate the mineral, fat, and mineral-free lean tissues of the body from x-ray attenuation.

essential lipids — Compound lipids (phospholipids) needed for cell membrane formation; approximately 10% of the total body lipid pool.

eumenorrhea — A normal menstrual cycle with 10 to 13 menstrual periods per year.

fat mass (FM) — All extractable lipids from adipose and other tissues in the body.

fat-free body (FFB) — All residual, lipid-free chemicals and tissues including water, muscle, bone, connective tissue, and internal organs.

fat-free body density (FFB_d) — The overall density of the water, mineral, and protein components of the fat-free body.

fat-free mass (FFM) — See fat-free body.

female triad — A pattern of disordered eating, amenorrhea, and premature osteoporosis characteristic of some female athletes.

FIT index — A crude measure of physical activity level based on subjective ratings of the frequency, intensity, and time (duration) of aerobic activity; scores range from 1 to 100.

generalized equations — Prediction equations used to estimate body composition of heterogeneous groups who vary greatly in age, gender, ethnicity, level of body fatness, and physical activity level.

gold standard — The method used in research settings to obtain reference measures of body composition (e.g., hydrodensitometry, neutron activation analysis).

gynoid obesity — Lower-body obesity; pear-shaped; accumulation of adipose tissue on the hips and thighs.

hydrodensitometry — A body composition method used to estimate body volume by measuring weight loss when the body is totally submerged under water.

impedance (Z) — A measure of the opposition to the flow of electrical current through the body; composed of two vectors—resistance and reactance.

intra-abdominal fat — Visceral fat in the abdominal cavity.

lean body mass (LBM) — The fat-free mass plus essential lipids.

line of best fit — The regression line depicting the relationship between the reference values and predicted body composition scores for a group of individuals.

line of identity — A straight line with a slope equal to 1 and an intercept equal to 0; used in a scatterplot to illustrate the differences in the measured and predicted scores of the cross-validation sample.

magnetic resonance imaging (MRI) — Technique used to create computerized cross-sectional images of the human body.

minimal body weight (MW) — The body weight corresponding to 5 %BF for males and 12 %BF for females.

multicomponent model — Body composition model that accounts for interindividual variation in the water, mineral, and protein content of the fat-free body.

multiple correlation coefficient (R_{mc}) — The correlation between the reference measure and predictor variables in the body composition equation.

multiple regression analysis — A statistical method used to derive and cross-validate body composition prediction equations.

near-infrared interactance (NIR) — A body composition method used to estimate percent body fat or total body density by measuring the reflectance of near-infrared light at the measurement site.

nomogram — A graph usually consisting of three parallel scales graduated for different variables so that when two values are plotted and connected by a straight line, the value of the third variable can be read directly at the point intersected by the line; used in body composition to calculate variables such as %BF, waist-to-hip ratio, and body mass index.

non-essential lipids — Triglycerides found primarily in adipose tissue; approximately 90% of the total-body lipid pool.

obesity — An excessive amount of total body fat for a given body weight; ≥ 25 %BF for men and ≥ 32 %BF for women.

optical density (OD) — A measure of the amount of near-infrared light reflected by the body's tissues at specific wavelengths (i.e., 940 and 950 nm).

osteoporosis — The loss of bone mineral content associated with aging, amenorrhea, malnutrition, or excessive exercise.

population-specific conversion formula — A formula used to convert Db to %BF for individuals from a specific population subgroup; formulas vary depending on the age, ethnicity, gender, level of body fatness, and physical activity level of the individual.

population-specific equations — Prediction equations used to estimate body composition of individuals from a specific homogenous group (e.g., children, athletes, or American Indians).

prediction equation — A mathematical formula derived from multiple regression analysis and used to estimate body composition measures (e.g., %BF, Db, and FFM).

prediction error — A measure of the predictive inaccuracy of a prediction equation in estimating reference measures of body composition (i.e., the standard error of estimate and total error).

predictor variables — Variables used to estimate the reference measure (e.g., %BF, FFM, Db) of body composition.

reactance (X_c) — A measure of opposition to current flow through the body due to the capacitance of cell membranes; a vector of impedance.

reference body — A theoretically and empirically derived body whose fat-free body is 73.8% water, 6.8% mineral, and 19.4% protein.

reference method — The "gold standard" body composition method used in research settings to develop and cross-validate body composition field methods and prediction equations (e.g., hydrodensitometry and neutron-activation analysis).

regression weight — A constant for each predictor variable in a body composition prediction equation; each predictor variable is multiplied by its constant and the products are summed to yield an estimate of the body composition measure being predicted.

relative body fat (%BF) — The fat mass expressed as a percentage of total body mass.

residual lung volume (RV) — The volume of air remaining in the lungs following a maximal expiration.

resistance (R) — A measure of pure opposition to the flow of electrical current flowing through the body; a vector of impedance; the lesser the resistance, the greater the current flow.

resistance index (HT^2/R) — Predictor variable in some BIA equations that is calculated by dividing height squared by total body resistance.

scatterplot — A graph used to illustrate the relationship between two variables.

skinfold (SKF) — A measure of the thickness of two layers of skin and the underlying subcutaneous fat.

sliding caliper — A small anthropometer used to measure the breadth of small body segments with a maximum measurement of 30 cm.

somatogram — An anthropometric profile that graphically depicts the body's pattern of muscle and fat distribution.

specific resistivity (p) — A constant physical property analogous to specific gravity; the reciprocal of conductance; assumed to be a constant value in most BIA models.

spreading caliper — An anthropometer shaped to allow measurement between anatomical landmarks that would be difficult to measure using a standard anthropometer (e.g., wrist and ankle breadths).

stadiometer — An instrument used to measure stature or standing height.

standard anthropometer — A narrow or broad-blade instrument used to measure the breadth and length of large body segments with a maximum measurement of 60-80 cm.

standard error of estimate (SEE) — A measure of the average deviation of individual scores from the regression line or line of best fit.

subcutaneous fat — Adipose tissue stored underneath the skin.

sum of skinfolds (ΣSKF) — The sum of two or more skinfold thicknesses.

supine — Back-lying body position.

total body mineral (TBM) — A measure of the osseous (bone) and non-osseous mineral content of the body.

total body water (TBW) — A measure of the intracellular and extracellular fluid compartments of the body.

total prediction error (E) — The average deviation of individual scores of the cross-validation sample from the line of identity.

two-component model — Body composition model that divides the body into fat and fat-free body components.

validity coefficient ($r_{y,y'}$) — The correlation between the measured and predicted scores of the cross-validation sample.

vernier caliper — A high precision instrument with a small, movable, graduated scale running parallel with a fixed, graduated scale of a ruler, providing highly precise and accurate linear measurements; used in body composition to calibrate skinfold calipers and small sliding calipers.

visceral fat — Adipose tissue within and around the organs in the thoracic and abdominal cavities.

waist-to-hip ratio (WHR) — The waist circumference divided by the hip circumference; used as a measure of upper-body or abdominal obesity.

References

Abraham, S., & Nordsieck, M. (1960). Relationship of excess weight in children and adults. *Public Health Reports*, **75**, 263-273.

Adams, P., Davies, G.T., & Sweetnam, P. (1970). Osteoporosis and the effects of aging on bone mineral mass in elderly men and women. *Quarterly Journal of Medicine*, **39**, 601-615.

Albu, S., Lichtman, S. Heymsfield, S., Wang, J., Pierson, R.N., & PiSunyer, F.X. (1989). Reassessment of body composition models in morbidly obese. *Federation of American Societies for Experimental Biology Journal*, **3**, A336.

Aloia, J.F., Cohn, S.H., Babu, T., Abesamis, C., Kalici, N., & Elllis, K. (1978). Skeletal mass and body composition in marathon runners. *Metabolism*, **27**, 1793-1796.

American College of Sports Medicine. (1985). *Position stand and opinion statements (1975-85)* (3rd ed.). Indianapolis, IN: Author.

American College of Sports Medicine. (1992). *The female athlete triad*. Indianapolis, IN: Author. (Slide presentation of Women's Task Force)

American Heart Association. (1994). 1995 *Heart and stroke facts statistics*. Dallas, TX: Author.

American Medical Association. (1967). Wrestling and weight control. *Journal of the American Medical Association*, **201**, 541-543.

American Psychiatric Association. (1994). *Diagnostic and statistical manual of mental disorders: IV* (4th ed.). Washington, D.C.: Author.

Ashwell, M., McCall, S.A., Cole, T.J., & Dixon, A.K. (1985). Fat distribution and its metabolic complications: Interpretations. In: N.G. Norgan (Ed.), *Human body composition and fat distribution* (pp. 227-242). Waginegen, Netherlands: Euronut.

Baumgartner, R.N., Chumlea, W.C., & Roche, A.F. (1988). Bioelectric impedance phase angle and body composition. *American Journal of Clinical Nutrition*, **48**, 16-23.

Baumgartner, R.N., Chumlea, W.C., & Roche, A.F. (1990). Bioelectrical impedance for body composition. *Exercise and Sport Sciences Reviews*, **18**, 193-224.

Baumgartner, R.N., Heymsfield, S.B., Lichtman, S., Wang, J., & Pierson, R.N. (1991). Body composition in elderly people: Effect of criterion estimates on predictive equations. *American Journal of Clinical Nutrition*, **53**, 1-9.

Baun, W.B., & Baun, M.R. (1981). A nomogram for the estimate of percent body fat from generalized equations. *Research Quarterly for Exercise and Sport, 52*, 380-384.

Behnke, A.R. (1961). Quantitative assessment of body build. *Journal of Applied Physiology, 16*, 960-968.

Behnke, A.R., & Wilmore, J.H. (1974). *Evaluation and regulation of body build and composition*. Englewood Cliffs, NJ: Prentice-Hall.

Belford, M., Stout, J., Eckerson, J., Housh, T., & Johnson, G. (1993). The validity of bioelectrical impedance, near-infrared interactance and skinfold equations for estimating body composition in females. *Medicine and Science in Sports and Exercise, 25*, S162. (Abstract)

Bjorntorp, P. (1985). Fat patterning and disease: A review. In N.G. Norgan (Ed.), *Human body composition and fat distribution* (pp. 201-209). Wageningen, Netherlands: Euronut.

Bjorntorp, P. (1988). Abdominal obesity and the development of non-insulin diabetes mellitus. *Diabetes and Metabolism Reviews, 4*, 615-622.

Bjorntorp, P. (1990). "Portal" adipose tissue as a generator of risk factors for cardiovascular disease and diabetes. *Atherosclerosis, 10*, 493-496.

Blair D., Habricht J.P., Sims, E.A., Sylwester D., & Abraham S. (1984). Evidence for an increased risk for hypertension with centrally located body fat, and the effect of race and sex on this risk. *American Journal of Epidemiology, 119*, 526-540.

Boileau, R.A., Lohman, T.G., & Slaughter, M.H. (1985). Exercise and body composition of children and youth. *Scandinavian Journal of Sports Science, 7*, 17-27.

Boileau, R.A., Lohman, T.G., Slaughter, M.H., Ball, T.E., Going, S.B., & Hendrix, M.K. (1984). Hydration of the fat-free body in children during maturation. *Human Biology, 56*, 651-666.

Boileau, R.A., Wilmore, J.H., Lohman, T.G., Slaughter, M.H., & Riner, W.F. (1981). Estimation of body density from skinfold thicknesses, body circumferences and skeletal widths in boys aged 8 to 11 years: Comparison of two samples. *Human Biology, 53*, 575-592.

Bray, G.A. (1978). Definitions, measurements and classifications of the syndromes of obesity. *International Journal of Obesity, 2*, 99-113.

Bray, G.A., & Gray, D.S. (1988a). Anthropometric measurements in the obese. In T.G. Lohman, A.F. Roche, & R. Martorell (Eds.), *Anthropometric standardization reference manual* (pp. 131-136). Champaign, IL: Human Kinetics.

Bray, G.A., & Gray, D.S. (1988b). Obesity. Part I--Pathogenesis. *Western Journal of Medicine, 149*, 429-441.

Bray, G.A., Greenway, F.L., Molitch, M.E., Dahms, W.T., Atkinson, R.L., & Hamilton, K. (1978). Use of anthropometric measures to assess weight loss. *American Journal of Clinical Nutrition, 31*, 769-773.

Broekhoff, C., Voorrips, L.E., Weijenberg, M.P., Witvoet, G.A., van Staveren, W.A., & Durenberg, P. (1992). Relative validity of different methods to assess body composition in apparently healthy elderly women. *Annals of Nutrition and Metabolism, 36*, 148-156.

Broussard, B.A., Johnson, A., Himes, J.H., Story, M., Fichtner, R., Hauck, F., Bachman-Carter, K., Hayes, J., Frohlich, K., Gray, N., Valway, S., & Gohdes, D. (1991). Prevalence of obesity in American Indians and Alaskan Natives. *American Journal of Clinical Nutrition, 53*, 1535S-1542S.

Brozek, J., Grande, F., Anderson, J.T., & Keys, A. (1963). Densitometric analysis of body composition: Revision of some quantitative assumptions. *Annals of the New York Academy of Sciences, 110*, 113-140.

Brozek, J., & Keys, A. (1951). Evaluation of leanness-fatness in man: Norms and interrelationships. *British Journal of Nutrition*, **5**, 194-206.

Bunt, J.C., Going, S.B., Lohman, T.G., Heinrich, C.H., Perry, C.D., & Pamenter, R.W. (1990). Variation in bone mineral content and estimated body fat in young adult females. *Medicine and Science in Sports and Exercise*, **22**, 564-569.

Bunt, J.C., Lohman, T.G., & Boileau, R.A. (1989). Impact of total body water fluctuations on estimation of body fat from body density. *Medicine and Science in Sports and Exercise*, **21**, 96-100.

Burgert, S.L., & Anderson, C.F. (1979). A comparison of triceps skinfold values as measured by the plastic McGaw caliper and the Lange caliper. *American Journal of Clinical Nutrition*, **32**, 1531-1533.

Busetto, L., Baggio, M.B., Zurlo F., Carraro R., Digito, M., & Enzi G. (1992). Assessment of abdominal fat distribution in obese patients: Anthropometry versus computerized tomography. *International Journal of Obesity*, **16**, 731-736.

Callaway, C.W., Chumlea, W.C., Bouchard, C., Himes, J.H., Lohman, T.G., Martin, A.D., Mitchell, C.D., Mueller, W.H., Roche, A.F., & Seefeldt, V.D. (1988). Circumferences. In T.G. Lohman, A.F. Roche, & R. Martorell (Eds.), *Anthropometric standardization reference manual* (pp. 39-54). Champaign, IL: Human Kinetics.

Carter Center of Emory University. (1985). Closing the gap: The problem of diabetes mellitus in the United States. *Diabetes Care*, **8**, 391-406.

Cassady, S.L., Nielsen, D.H., Janz, K.F., Wu, Y., Cook, J.S., & Hansen, J.R. (1993). Validity of near infrared body composition analysis in children and adolescents. *Medicine and Science in Sports and Exercise*, **25**, 1185-1191.

Caton, J.R., Mole, P.A., Adams, W.C., & Heustis, D.S. (1988). Body composition analysis by bioelectrical impedance: Effect of skin temperature. *Medicine and Science in Sports and Exercise*, **20**, 489-491.

Charney, E., Goodman, H.C., McBridge, M., Lyon, B., & Pratt, R. (1976). Childhood antecedents of adult obesity: Do chubby infants become obese adults? *The New England Journal of Medicine*, **295**, 6-9.

Chumlea, W.C., & Baumgartner, R.N. (1989). Status of anthropometry and body composition data in elderly subjects. *American Journal of Clinical Nutrition*, **50**, 1158-1166.

Chumlea, W.C., Baumgartner, R.N., & Roche, A.F. (1988). Specific resistivity used to estimate fat-free mass from segmental body measures of bioelectric impedance. *American Journal of Clinical Nutrition*, **48**, 7-15.

Clark, R.R., Kuta, J.M., & Sullivan, J.C. (1993). Prediction of percent body fat in adult males using dual energy x-ray absorptiometry, skinfolds, and hydrostatic weighing. *Medicine and Science in Sports and Exercise*, **25**, 528-535.

Clark, R.R., Kuta, J.M., Sullivan, J.C., Bedford, W.M., Penner, J.D., & Studesville, E.A. (1993). A comparison of methods to predict minimal weight in high school wrestlers. *Medicine and Science in Sports and Exercise*, **25**, 151-158.

Clarys, J.P., Martin, A.D., Drinkwater, D.T., & Marfell-Jones, M.J. (1987). The skinfold: Myth and reality. *Journal of Sports Sciences*, **5**, 3-33.

Cohn, S.H., Abesamis, C., Zanzi, I., Aloia, J.F., Yasumura, S., & Ellis, K.J. (1977). Body elemental composition: Comparison between black and white adults. *American Journal of Physiology*, **232**(4), E419-E422.

Colville, B.C., Heyward, V.H., & Sandoval, W.M. (1989). Comparison of two methods for estimating body composition of bodybuilders. *Journal of Applied Sport Science Research*, **3**, 57-61.

Conway, J.M., & Norris, K.H. (1987). Noninvasive body composition in humans by near infrared interactance. In K.J. Ellis, S. Yasumura, & W.D. Morgan (Eds.), *In vivo body composition studies* (pp. 163-170). Brookhaven, NY: The Institute of Physical Sciences in Medicine.

Conway, J.M., Norris, K.H., & Bodwell, C.E. (1984). A new approach for the estimation of body composition: Infrared interactance. *American Journal of Clinical Nutrition, 40*, 1123-1130.

Curb, J.D., & Marcus, E.B. (1991). Body fat and obesity in Japanese Americans. *American Journal of Clinical Nutrition, 53*, 1552S-1555S.

Damon, A. (1965). Notes on anthropometric technique: II. Skinfolds--right and left sides: held by one or two hands. *American Journal of Physical Anthropology, 23*, 305-306.

Davis, P.G., Van Loan, M., Holly, R.G., Krstich, K., & Phinney, S.D. (1989). Near infrared interactance vs. hydrostatic weighing to measure body composition in lean, normal, and obese women. *Medicine and Science in Sports and Exercise, 21*, S100. (Abstract)

Davis, P.O., Dotson, C.O., & Manny, P.D. (1988). NIR evaluation for body composition analysis. *Medicine and Science in Sports and Exercise, 20*, S8. (Abstract)

Deck-Cote, K., & Adams, W.C. (1993). Effect of bone density on body composition estimates in young adult black and white women. *Medicine and Science in Sports and Exercise, 25*, 290-296.

Dempsey, D.T., Crosby, L.O., Lusk, E., Oberlander, J.L., Pertschuk, M.J., & Mullen, J.L. (1984). Total body water and total body potassium in anorexia nervosa. *American Journal of Clinical Nutrition, 40*, 260-269.

Despres, J.P. (1991). Lipoprotein metabolism in visceral obesity. *International Journal of Obesity, 15*, 45-52.

Despres, J.P., Fong, B.S., Julien, P., Jimenez, J., & Angel, A. (1987). Regional variation in HDL metabolism in human fat cells: Effect of fat cell size. *American Journal of Physiology, 252*, E654-E659.

Despres, J.P., Prud'homme, D., Pouliot, M.C., Tremblay, A., & Bouchard C. (1991). Estimation of deep abdominal adipose-tissue accumulation from simple anthropometric measurements in men. *American Journal of Clinical Nutrition, 54*, 471-477.

Deurenberg, P., Kusters, C.S., & Smit, H.E. (1990). Assessment of body composition by bioelectrical impedance in children and young adults is strongly age-dependent. *European Journal of Clinical Nutrition, 44*, 261-268.

Deurenberg, P., Leenan, R., van der Kooy, K., & Hautvast, J.G. (1989). In obese subjects the body fat percentage calculated with Siri's formula is an overestimation. *European Journal of Clinical Nutrition, 43*, 569-575.

Deurenberg, P., van der Kooy, K., Evers, P., & Hulshof, T. (1990). Assessment of body composition by bioelectrical impedance in a population aged > 60 y. *American Journal of Clincial Nutrtion, 51*, 3-6.

Deurenberg, P., van der Kooy, K., & Leenan, R. (1989). Differences in body impedance when measured with different instruments. *European Journal of Clinical Nutrition, 43*, 885-886.

Deurenberg, P., van der Kooy, K., Leenan, R., Weststrate, J.A., & Seidell, J.C. (1991). Sex and age specific population prediction formulas for estimating body composition from bioelectrical impedance: A cross-validation study. *International Journal of Obesity, 15*, 17-25.

Deurenberg, P., Weststrate, J.A., & Hautvast, J.G. (1989). Changes in fat-free mass during weight loss measured by bioelectrical impedance and by densitometry. *American Journal of Clinical Nutrition, 49*, 33-36.

Deurenberg, P., Weststrate, J.A., Hautvast, J.G., & van der Kooy, K. (1991). Is the bioelectrical-impedance method valid? *American Journal of Clinical Nutrition, 53*, 179. (Letter to editor)

Deurenberg, P., Weststrate, J.A., Paymans, I., & van der Kooy, K. (1988). Factors affecting bioelectrical impedance measurements in humans. *European Journal of Clincal Nutrition, 42*, 1017-1022.

Deurenberg. P., Westrate, J.A., & Seidell, J.C. (1991). Body mass index as a measure of body fatness: Age- and sex-specific prediction formulas. *British Journal of Nutrition, 65*, 105-114.

Deurenberg, P., Westrate, J.A., & van der Kooy, K. (1989a). Body composition changes assessed by bioelectrical impedance measurements. *American Journal of Clinical Nutrition, 49*, 401-403.

Deurenberg. P., Westrate, J.A., & van der Kooy, K. (1989b). Is an adaptation of Siri's formula for the calculation of body fat percentage from body density in the elderly necessary? *European Journal of Clinical Nutrition, 43*, 559-568.

DeWaart, F.G., Li, R., & Deurenberg, P. (1993). Comparison of body composition assessments by bioelectrical impedance and by anthropometry in premenopausal Chinese women. *British Journal of Nutrition, 69*, 657-664.

Donahue R.P., Abbot R.D., Bloom E., Reed D.M., & Yano K. (1987). Central fat distribution in middle-aged men and the risk of coronary heart disease in men. *Lancet, 1*, 822-824.

Drinkwater, B.L., Nilson, K., Chesnut, C.H., Bremner, W.J., Shainholtz, S., & Southworth, M.B. (1984). Bone mineral content of amenorrheic and eumenorrheic athletes. *The New England Journal of Medicine, 311*, 277-281.

Ducimetier P., Richard J., & Cambien F. (1989). The pattern of subcutaneous fat distribution in middle-aged men and the risk of coronary heart disease: The Paris prospective study. *International Journal of Obesity, 10*, 229-240.

Durnin, J.V., & Rahamen, M.M. (1967). The assessment of the amount of fat in the human body from measurements of skinfold thickness. *British Journal of Nutrition, 21*, 681-689.

Durnin, J.V., & Womersley, J. (1974). Body fat assessed from body density and its estimation from skinfold thickness: Measurements on 481 men and women aged from 16 to 72 years. *British Journal of Nutrition, 32*, 77-97.

Eaton, A.W., Israel, R.G., O'Brien, K.F., Hortobagyi, T., & McCammon, M.R. (1993). Comparison of four methods to assess body composition in women. *European Journal of Clinical Nutrition, 47*, 353-360.

Eckerson, J.M., Housh, T.J., & Johnson, G.O. (1992). Validity of bioelectrical impedance equations for estimating fat-free weight in lean males. *Medicine and Science in Sports and Exercise, 24*, 1298-1302.

Edwards, D.A., Hammond, W.H., Healy, M.J., Tanner, J.M., & Whitehouse, R.H. (1955). Design and accuracy of calipers for measuring subcutaneous tissue thickness. *British Journal of Nutrition, 9*, 133-143.

Elia, M., Parkinson, S.A., & Diaz, E. (1990). Evaluation of near infra-red interactance as a method for predicting body composition. *European Journal of Clinical Nutrition, 44*, 113-121.

Elsen, R., Siu, M.L., Pineda, O., & Solomons, N.W. (1987). Sources of variability in bioelectrical impedance determinations in adults. In K.J. Ellis, S. Yasamura, & W.D. Morgan (Eds.), *In vivo body composition studies* (pp. 184-188). London: The Institute of Physical Sciences in Medicine.

Espejo, M.G.A., Neu, J., Hamilton, L., Eitzman, B., Gimotty, P., & Bucciarelli, R.L. (1989). Determination of extracellular fluid volume using impedance measurements. *Critical Care Medicine, 17*, 360-363.

Ferland, M., Despres, J.P., Tremblay, A., Pinault, S., Nadeau, A., Moorjani, S., Lupien, P.J., Theriault, G., & Bouchard C. (1989). Assessment of adipose distribution by computed axial tomography in obese women: Association with body density and anthropometric measurements. *British Journal of Nutrition, 61*, 139-148.

Fleck, S.J. (1983). Body composition of elite American athletes. *American Journal of Sports Medicine, 11*, 398-403.

Fohlin, L. (1977). Body composition, cardiovascular and renal function in adolescent patients with anorexia nervosa. *Acta Paediatrica Scandinavica, 268*(Suppl.), 7-20.

Folsom, A.R., Burke, G.L., Byers, C.L., Hutchinson, R.G., Heiss, G., Flack, J.M., Jacobs, D.R., & Caan, B. (1991). Implications of obesity for cardiovascular disease in blacks: The CARDIA and ARIC studies. *American Journal of Clinical Nutrition, 53*, 1604S-1611S.

Fomon, S.J., Haschke, F., Ziegler, E.E. & Nelson, S.E. (1982). Body composition of reference children from birth to age 10 years. *American Journal of Clinical Nutrition, 35*, 1169-1175.

Forbes, G.B., Simon, W., & Amatruda, J.M. (1992). Is bioimpedance a good predictor of body-composition change? *American Journal of Clinical Nutrition, 56*, 4-6.

Forsyth, H.L., & Sinning, W.E. (1973). The anthropometric estimation of body density and lean body weight of male athletes. *Medicine and Science in Sports, 5*, 174-180.

Franzen, R. (1929). *Physical measures of growth and nutrition.* New York: American Child Health Association.

Fredrix, E.W., Saris, W.H., Soeters, P.B., Wouters, E.F., Kester, A.D., von Meyenfeldt, M.F., & Westerterp, K.R. (1990). Estimation of body composition by bioelectrical impedance in cancer patients. *European Journal of Clinical Nutrition, 44*, 749-752.

Friedl, K.E., DeLuca, J.P., Marchitelli, L.J., & Vogel, J.A. (1992). Reliability of body-fat estimations from a four-compartment model by using density, body water, and bone mineral measurements. *American Journal of Clinical Nutrition, 55*, 764-770.

Frisancho, A.R. (1984). New standard of weight and body composition by frame size and height for assessment of nutritional status of adults and the elderly. *American Journal of Clincial Nutrition, 40*, 808-819.

Frisancho, A.R., & Flegel, P.N. (1983). Elbow breadth as a measure of frame size for US males and females. *American Journal of Clinical Nutrition, 37*, 311-314.

Fulcher, G.R., Farrer, M., Walker, M., Rodham, D., Clayton, B., & Alberti, G.M.M. (1991). A comparison of measurements of lean body mass derived by bioelectrical impedance, skinfold thickness and total body potassium. A study in obese and non-obese normal subjects. *Scandinavian Journal of Clinical and Laboratory Investigation, 51*, 245-253.

Fuller, N.J., & Elia, M. (1989). Potential use of bioelectrical impedance of "whole body" and of body segments for the assessment of body composition: A comparison with densitometry and anthropometry. *European Journal of Clinical Nutrition, 43*, 779-791.

Fuller, N.J., Jebb, S.A., Laskey, M.A., Coward, W.A., & Elia, M. (1992). Four-component model for the assessment of body composition in humans: Comparison with alternative methods, and evaluation of the density and hydration of fat-free mass. *Clinical Science, 82*, 687-693.

Futrex, Inc. (1988). *Futrex-5000 Research Manual.* Gaithersburg, MD. Author.

Garn, S.M., Leonard, W.R., & Hawthorne, V.M. (1986). Three limitations of the body mass index. *American Journal of Clinical Nutrition, 44*, 996-997.

Garrow, J.S., & Webster, J. (1985). Quetelet's index (W/H²) as a measure of fatness. *International Journal of Obesity, 9*, 147-153.

Gaskill, S.P., Allen, C.R., Garza, V., Gonzales, J.L., & Waldrop, R.H. (1981) Cardiovascular risk factors in Mexican-Americans in Laredo, Texas. I. Prevalence of overweight and diabetes and distribution of serum lipids. *American Journal of Epidemiology, 113*, 546-555.

George, C.M., Wells, C.L., & Dugan, N.L. (1988). Validity of hydrodensitometry for determination of body composition in spinal injured subjects. *Human Biology, 60*, 771-780.

Gleichauf, C.N., & Rose, D.A. (1989). The menstrual cycle's effect on the reliability of bioimpedance measurements for assessing body composition. *American Journal of Clinical Nutrition, 50*, 903-907.

Going, S.B., & Lohman, T.G. (1990). The skinfold test--A response. *Journal of Physical Education, Recreation, and Dance, 61*, 74-78.

Going, S.B., Lohman, T.G., Williams, D.P., Hewitt, M.J., & Haber, A. (1989). Prediction of trunk soft tissue composition from trunk bioelectrical impedance analysis in older men and women. *Medicine and Science in Sports and Exercise, 21*, S39. (Abstract)

Going, S.B., Massett, M.P., Hall, M.C., Bare, L.A., Root, P.A., Williams, D.P., & Lohman, T.G. (1993). Detection of small changes in body composition by dual-energy x-ray absorptiometry. *American Journal of Clinical Nutrition, 57*, 845-850.

Gomez, T., Mole, P.A., & Collins, A. (1993). Dilution of body fluid electrolytes affects bioelectrical impedance measurements. *Sports Medicine, Training, and Rehabilitation, 4*, 291-298.

Gordon, C.C., Chumlea, W.C., & Roche, A.F. (1988). Stature, recumbent length, and weight. In T.G. Lohman, A.F. Roche, & R. Martorell (Eds.), *Anthropometric standardization reference manual* (pp. 3-8), Champaign, IL: Human Kinetics.

Grant, J.P., Custer, P.B., & Thurlaw, J. (1981). Current techniques of nutritional assessment. *Surgical Clinics of North America, 61*, 437-463.

Graves, J.E., Pollock, M.L., Colvin, A.B., Van Loan, M., & Lohman, T.G. (1989). Comparison of different bioelectrical impedance analyzers in the prediction of body composition. *American Journal of Human Biology, 1*, 603-611.

Gray, D.S., Bray, G.A., Bauer, M., Kaplan, K., Gemayel, N., Wood, R., Greenway, R., & Kirk, S. (1990). Skinfold thickness measurements in obese subjects. *American Journal of Clinical Nutrition, 51*, 571-577.

Gray, D.S., Bray, G.A., Gemayel, N., & Kaplan, K. (1989). Effect of obesity on bioelectrical impedance. *American Journal of Clinical Nutrition, 50*, 255-260.

Gray, D.S., & Fujioka, K. (1991). Use of relative weight and body mass index for the determination of adiposity. *Journal of Clinical Epidemiology, 44*, 545-550.

Gruber, J.J., Pollock, M.L., Graves, J.E., Colvin, A.B., & Braith, R.W. (1990). Comparison of Harpenden and Lange calipers in predicting body composition. *Research Quarterly for Exercise and Sport, 61*, 184-190.

Guo, S., Roche, A.F., & Houtkooper, L. (1989). Fat-free mass in children and young adults predicted from biotechnic impedance and anthropometric variables. *American Journal of Clincial Nutrition, 50,* 435-443.

Haffner, S.M., Stern, M.P., Mitchell, B.D., Hazuda, H.P., & Patterson, J.K. (1990). Incidence of type II diabetes in Mexican-Americans predicted by fasting insulin and glucose levels, obesity, and body-fat distribution. *Diabetes, 39,* 283-288.

Hagiwara, S., Miki, T., Nishizawa, Y., Ochi, H., Onoyama, Y., & Morii, H. (1989). Quantification of bone mineral content using dual-photon absorptiometry in normal Japanese population. *Journal of Bone and Mineral Research, 4,* 217-222.

Hansen, N.J., Lohman, T.G., Going, S.B., Hall, M.C., Pamenter, R.W., Bare, L.A., Boyden, T.W., & Houtkooper, L.B. (1993). Prediction of body composition in premenopausal females from dual-energy x-ray absorptiometry. *Journal of Applied Physiology, 75,* 1637-1641.

Harrison, G.G., Buskirk, E.R., Lindsay Carter, J.E., Johnston, F.E., Lohman, T.G., Pollock, M.L., Roche, A.F., & Wilmore, J.H. (1988). Skinfold thicknesses and measurement technique. In T.G. Lohman, A.F. Roche, & R. Martorell (Eds.), *Anthropometric standardization reference manual* (pp. 55-70). Champaign, IL: Human Kinetics.

Harsha, D.W., Frerichs, R.R., & Berenson, G.S. (1978). Densitometry and anthropometry of black and white children. *Human Biology, 50,* 261-280.

Hart, P.D., Wilkie, M.E., Edwards, A., & Cunningham, J. (1993). Dual energy x-ray absorptiometry versus skinfold measurements in the assessment of total body fat in renal transplant recipients. *European Journal of Clinical Nutrition, 47,* 347-352.

Haschke, F. (1983). Body composition of adolescent males. Part II. Body composition of the male reference adolescent. *Acta Paediatrica Scandinavica, 307*(Suppl.), 11-23.

Hawkins, J.D. (1983). An analysis of selected skinfold measuring instruments. *Journal of Health, Physical Education, Recreation, and Dance, 54,* 25-27.

Hayes, P.A., Sowood, P.J., Belyavin, A., Cohen, J.B., & Smith, F.W. (1988). Subcutaneous fat thickness measured by magnetic resonance imaging, ultrasound, and calipers. *Medicine and Science in Sports and Exercise, 20,* 303-309.

Heitmann, B.L. (1990). Prediction of body water and fat in adult Danes from measurement of electrical impedance. A validation study. *International Journal of Obesity, 14,* 789-802.

Hergenroeder, A.C., Brown, B., & Klish, W.J. (1993). Anthropometric measurements and estimating body composition in ballet dancers. *Medicine and Science in Sports and Exercise, 25,* 145-150.

Heymsfield, S.B., Lichtman, S., Baumgartner, R.N., Wang, J., Kamen, Y., Aliprantis, A., & Pierson, R.N. (1990). Body composition of humans: Comparison of two improved four-compartment models that differ in expense, technical complexity, and radiation exposure. *American Journal of Clinical Nutrition, 52,* 52-58.

Heymsfield, S.B., Wang, J., Lichtman, S., Kamen, Y., Kehayias, J., & Pierson, R.N. (1989). Body composition in elderly subjects: A critical appraisal of clinical methodology. *American Journal of Clinical Nutrition, 50,* 1167-1175.

Heyward, V.H., Cook, K.L., Hicks, V.L., Jenkins, K.A., Quatrochi, J.A. & Wilson, W. (1992). Predictive accuracy of three field methods for estimating relative body fatness of nonobese and obese women. *International Journal of Sport Nutrition, 2,* 75-86.

Heyward, V.H., Jenkins, K.A., Cook, K.L., Hicks, V.L., Quatrochi, J.A., Wilson, W., & Going, S. (1992). Validity of single-site and multi-site models of estimating body composition of women using near-infrared interactance. *American Journal of Human Biology,* **4**, 579-593.

Heyward, V.H., Jenkins, K.A., Mermier, C.M., & Stolarczyk, L. (1993). Sources of variability for optical density measures. *Medicine and Science in Sports and Exercise,* **25**, S60. (Abstract)

Heyward, V.H., Stolarczyk, L., Goodman, J., Grant, J., Kessler, K., Kocina, P., & Wilmerding, V. (1994, November). *Predictive accuracy of skinfold (SKF) and near-infrared interactance (NIR) equations in estimating body density of Hispanic women.* Presented at Southwest Regional meeting of American College of Sports Medicine, San Diego, CA.

Heyward, V.H., Wilson, W.L., & Stolarczyk, L.M. (1994). Predictive accuracy of BIA equations for estimating fat-free mass of American Indian, Black, and Hispanic men. *Medicine and Science in Sports and Exercise,* **26**, S202. (Abstract)

Hicks, V.L. (1992). *Validation of near-infrared interactance and skinfold methods for estimating body composition of American Indian women.* Unpublished doctoral dissertation, University of New Mexico, Albuquerque.

Hicks, V.L., Heyward, V.H., Baumgartner, R.N., Flores, A.J., Stolarczyk, L.M., & Wotruba, E.A. (1993). Body composition of Native American women estimated by dual-energy x-ray absorptiometry and hydrodensitometry. In K.J. Ellis, & J.D. Eastman (Eds.), *Human body composition: In vivo methods, models and assessment* (pp. 89-92). New York: Plenum.

Hicks, V., Heyward, V., Flores, A., Stolarczyk, L., Koppy, P., & Wotruba, E. (1993). Validation of near-infrared interactance (NIR) and skinfold (SKF) methods for estimating body composition of American Indian women. *Medicine and Science in Sports and Exercise,* **25**, S152. (Abstract)

Hicks, V.L., Wilson, W.L., & Heyward, V.H. (1992). Accuracy of bioelectrical impedance in estimating body composition of American Indians. *Medicine and Science in Sports and Exercise,* **24**, S6. (Abstract)

Himes, J.H., & Bouchard, C. (1985). Do the new metropolitan life insurance weight-height tables correctly assess body frame and body fat relationships? *American Journal of Public Health,* **75**, 1076-1079.

Himes, J.H., & Frisancho, R.A. (1988). Estimating frame size. In T.G. Lohman, A.F. Roche, & R. Martorell (Eds.), *Anthropometric standardization reference manual* (pp. 121-124). Champaign, IL: Human Kinetics.

Hodgdon, J.A. (1992). Body composition in the military services: Standards and methods. In B.M. Marriott, & J. Grumstrup-Scott (Eds.), *Body composition and physical performance: Applications for the military services* (pp. 57-70). Washington, DC: National Academy Press.

Hodgdon, J.A., & Fitzgerald, P.I. (1987). Validity of impedance predictions at various levels of fatness. *Human Biology,* **59**, 281-298.

Hoffer, E.C., Meador, C.K., & Simpson, D.C. (1969). Correlation of whole-body impedance with total body water volume. *Journal of Applied Physiology,* **27**, 531-534.

Horswill, C.A., Lohman, T.G., Slaughter, M.H., Boileau, R.A., & Wilmore, J.H. (1990). Estimation of minimal weight of adolescent males using multicomponent models. *Medicine and Science in Sports and Exercise,* **22**, 528-532.

Hortobagyi, T., Israel, R.G., Houmard, J.A., McCammon, M.R., & O'Brien, K.F. (1992). Comparison of body composition assessment by hydrodensitometry, skinfolds, and multiple site near-infrared spectrophotometry. *European Journal of Clinical Nutrition,* **46**, 205-211.

Hortobagyi, T., Israel, R.G., Houmard, J.A., O'Brien, K.F., Johns, R.A., & Wells, J.M. (1992). Comparison of four methods to assess body composition in black and white athletes. *International Journal of Sport Nutrition*, **2**, 60-74.

Houmard, J.A., Israel, R.G., McCammon, M.R., O'Brien, K.F., Omer, J., & Zamora, B.S. (1991). Validity of a near-infrared device for estimating body composition in a college football team. *Journal of Applied Sport Science Research*, **5**, 53-59.

Houtkooper, L.B., Going, S.B., Lohman, T.G., Roche, A.F., & Van Loan, M. (1992). Bioelectrical impedance estimation of fat-free body mass in children and youth: A cross-validation study. *Journal of Applied Physiology*, **72**, 366-373.

Houtkooper, L.B., Going, S.B., Westfall, C.H., & Lohman, T.G. (1989). Prediction of fat-free body corrected for bone mass from impedance and anthropometry in adult females. *Medicine and Science in Sports and Exercise*, **21**, S39. (Abstract)

Houtkooper, L.B., Lohman, T.G., Going, S.B., & Hall, M.C. (1989). Validity of bioelectric impedance for body composition assessment in children. *Journal of Applied Physiology*, **66**, 814-821.

Israel, R.G., Houmard, J.A., O'Brien, K.F., McCammon, M.R., Zamora, B.S., & Eaton, A.W. (1989). Validity of near-infrared spectrophotometry device for estimating human body composition. *Research Quarterly for Exercise and Sport*, **60**, 379-383.

Jackson, A. (1984). Research design and analysis of data procedures for predicting body density. *Medicine and Science in Sports and Exercise*, **16**, 616-620.

Jackson, A.S., & Pollock, M.L. (1976). Factor analysis and multivariate scaling of anthropometric variables for the assessment of body composition. *Medicine and Science in Sports and Exercise*, **8**, 196-203.

Jackson, A.S., & Pollock, M.L. (1978). Generalized equations for predicting body density of men. *British Journal of Nutrition*, **40**, 497-504.

Jackson, A.S., & Pollock, M.L. (1985). Practical assessment of body composition. *The Physician and Sportsmedicine*, **13**, 76-90.

Jackson, A.S., Pollock, M.L., Graves, J.E., & Mahar, M.T. (1988). Reliability and validity of bioelectrical impedance in determining body composition. *Journal of Applied Physiology*, **64**, 529-534.

Jackson, A.S., Pollock, M.L., & Ward, A. (1980). Generalized equations for predicting body density of women. *Medicine and Science in Sports and Exercise*, **12**, 175-182.

Jakicic, J.M., Donnelly, J.E., Jawad, A.F., Jacobsen, D.J., Gunderson, S.C., & Pascale R. (1993). Association between blood lipids and different measures of body fat distribution: Effects of BMI and age. *International Journal of Obesity*, **17**, 131-137.

Janz, K.F., Nielsen, D.H., Cassady, S.L., Cook, J.S., Wu, Y., & Hansen, J.R. (1993). Cross-validation of the Slaughter skinfold equations for children and adolescents. *Medicine and Science in Sports and Exercise*, **25**, 1070-1076.

Jenkins, K.A., Heyward, V.H., Cook, K.L., Hicks, V.L., Quatrochi, J.A., Wilson, W.L. & Colville, B.C. (1994). Predictive accuracy of bioelectrical impedance equations for women. *American Journal of Human Biology*, **6**, 293-303.

Kahn, H.S. (1991). A major error in nomograms for estimating body mass index. *American Journal of Clinical Nutrition*, **54**, 435-437.

Kasari, D. (1976). *The Effects of Exercise and Fitness on Serum Lipids in College Women.* Unpublished master's thesis, University of Montana, Missoula, MT.

Katch, F.I., & Katch, V.L. (1980). Measurement and prediction errors in body composition assessment and the search for the perfect equation. *Research Quarterly for Exercise and Sport*, **51**, 249-260.

Katch, F.I., & McArdle, W.D. (1973). Prediction of body density from simple anthropometric measurements in college-age men and women. *Human Biology, 45*, 445-454.

Keteyian, S.J., Marks, C.R., Fedel, F.J., Ehrman, J.K., Goslin, B.R., Connolly, A.M., Fachnie, J.D., Levine, T.B., & O'Neil, M.J. (1992). Assessment of body composition in heart transplant patients. *Medicine and Science in Sports and Exercise, 24*, 247-252.

Keys, A., & Brozek, J. (1953). Body fat in adult man. *Physiological Reviews, 33*, 245-325.

Keys, A., Fidanza, F., Karvonen, M., Kimura, N., & Taylor, H.L. (1972). Indices of relative weight and obesity. *Journal of Chronic Diseases, 25*, 329-343.

Khaled, M.A., McCutcheon, M.J., Reddy, S., Pearman, P.L. Hunter, G.R., & Weinsier, R.L. (1988). Electrical impedance in assessing human body composition: The BIA method. *American Journal of Clinical Nutrition, 47*, 789-792.

Kim, H.K., Tanaka, K., Nakadomo, F., Watanabe, K., & Matsuura, Y. (1993). Fat-free mass in Japanese boys predicted from bioelectrical impedance and anthropometric variables. *Medicine and Science in Sports and Exercise, 25*, S59. (Abstract)

Kin, K., Lee, J.H.E., Kushida, K., Ohmura, A., Inoue, T., Clopton, P., & Sartoris, D.J. (1992, November). *Total body composition and bone mineral density: A comparison between Japanese-American and Native Japanese women*. Paper presented at International Symposium for In Vivo Body Composition Studies, Houston, TX. (Abstract)

Klimis-Tavantis, D., Oulare, M., Lehnhard, H., & Cook, R.A. (1992). Near-infrared interactance: Validity and use in estimating body composition of adolescents. *Nutrition Research, 12*, 427-439.

Knowler, W.C., Pettitt, D.J., Savage, P.J., Bennett, P.H. (1981). Diabetes incidence in Pima Indians: Contributions of obesity and parental diabetes. *American Journal of Epidemiology, 113*, 144-156.

Kuczmarski, R.J. (1989). Need for body composition information in elderly subjects. *American Journal of Clinical Nutrition, 50*, 1150-1157.

Kuczmarski, R.J. (1992). Prevalence of overweight and weight gain in the United States. *American Journal of Clinical Nutrition, 55*, 495S-502S.

Kuczmarski, R.J., Flegal, K.M., Campbell, S.M., & Johnson, C.L. (1994). Increasing prevalence of overweight among U.S. adults: the National Health and Nutrition Examination Surveys, 1960 to 1991. *Journal of the American Medical Association, 272*, 205-211.

Kushner, R.F. (1992). Bioelectrical impedance analysis: A review of principles and applications. *Journal of the American College of Nutrition, 11*, 199-209.

Kushner, R.F., Kunigk, A., Alspaugh, M., Andronis, P.T., Leitch, C.A., & Schoeller, D.A. (1990). Validation of bioelectrical-impedance analysis as a measurement of change in body composition in obesity. *American Journal of Clinical Nutrition, 52*, 219-223.

Kushner, R.F., & Schoeller, D.A. (1986). Estimation of total body water in bioelectrical impedance analysis. *American Journal of Clinical Nutrition, 44*, 417-424.

Kushner, R.F., Schoeller, D.A., Fjeld, C.R., & Danford, L. (1992). Is the impedance index (ht^2/R) significant in predicting total body water? *American Journal of Clinical Nutrition, 56*, 835-839.

Larsson, B., Svardsudd, K., Welin, L., Wilhemsen, L., Bjorntorp, P. & Tibblin, G. (1984). Abdominal adipose tissue distribution, obesity and risk of cardiovascular disease and death: 13 year follow-up of participants in the study of men born in 1913. *British Medical Journal, 288*, 1401-1404.

Lee, J., & Hinds, M.W.(1981). Relative merits of the weight-corrected-for-height indices. *American Journal of Clinical Nutrition, 34*, 2521-2529.

Leger, L.A., Lambert, J., & Martin, P. (1982). Validity of plastic skinfold caliper measurements. *Human Biology, 54*, 667-675.

Lindsay, R., Cosman, F., Herrington, B.S., & Himmelstein, S. (1992). Bone mass and body composition in normal women. *Journal of Bone and Mineral Research, 7*, 55-63.

Lohman, T.G. (1981). Skinfolds and body density and their relation to body fatness: A review. *Human Biology, 53*, 181-225.

Lohman, T.G. (1986). Applicability of body composition techniques and constants for children and youth. In K.B. Pandolf (Ed.), *Exercise and sport sciences reviews* (pp. 325-357). New York: Macmillan.

Lohman, T.G. (1987). *Measuring body fat using skinfolds* [videotape]. Champaign, IL: Human Kinetics.

Lohman, T.G. (1989a). Assessment of body composition in children. *Pediatric Exercise Science, 1*, 19-30.

Lohman, T.G. (1989b). Bioelectrical impedance. In *Applying new technology to nutrition: Report of the ninth roundtable on medical issues* (pp. 22-25). Columbus, OH: Ross Laboratories.

Lohman, T.G. (1992). *Advances in body composition assessment.* Current issues in exercise science series. Monograph No.3. Champaign, IL: Human Kinetics.

Lohman, T.G., Boileau, R.A., & Slaughter, M.H. (1984). Body composition in children and youth. In R.A. Boileau (Ed.), *Advances in pediatric sport sciences* (pp. 29-57). Champaign, IL: Human Kinetics.

Lohman, T.G., Going, S.B., & Houtkooper, L.B. (1988). Body composition changes with training and various methods of estimating changes. *Report of the Ross Symposium on Muscle Development: Nutritional Alternatives to Anabolic Steroids* (pp. 22-26). Columbus, OH: Ross Laboratories.

Lohman, T.G., Pollock, M.L., Slaughter, M.H., Brandon, L.J., & Boileau, R.A. (1984). Methodological factors and the prediction of body fat in female athletes. *Medicine and Science in Sports and Exercise, 16*, 92-96.

Lohman, T.G., Roche, A.F., & Martorell, R. (Eds.) (1988). *Anthropometric standardization reference manual.* Champaign, IL: Human Kinetics.

Lohman, T.G., Slaughter, M.H., Boileau, R.A., Bunt, J., & Lussier, L. (1984). Bone mineral measurements and their relation to body density in children, youth, and adults. *Human Biology, 56*, 667-679.

Lukaski, H.C. (1986). Use of the tetrapolar bioelectrical impedance method to assess human body composition. In N.G. Norgan (Ed.), *Human body composition and fat patterning* (pp. 143-158). Waginegen, Netherlands: Euronut.

Lukaski, H.C. (1987). Methods for the assessment of human body composition: Traditional and new. *American Journal of Clinical Nutrition, 46*, 537-556.

Lukaski, H.C., & Bolonchuk, W.W. (1987). Theory and validation of the tetrapolar bioelectrical impedance method to assess human body composition. In K.J. Ellis, S. Yasamura, & W.D. Morgan (Eds.), *In vivo body composition studies* (pp. 410-414). London: The Institute of Physical Sciences in Medicine.

Lukaski, H.C., & Bolonchuk, W.W. (1988). Estimation of body fluid volumes using tetrapolar impedance measurements. *Aviation, Space, and Environmental Medicine, 59*, 1163-1169.

Lukaski, H.C., Bolonchuk, W.W., Hall, C.B., & Siders, W.A. (1986). Validation of tetrapolar bioelectrical impedance method to assess human body composition. *Journal of Applied Physiology, 60*, 1327-1332.

Lukaski, H.C., Bolonchuk, W.W., Siders, W.A., & Hall, C.B. (1990). Body composition assessment of athletes using bioelectrical impedance measurements. *Journal of Sports Medicine and Physical Fitness*, **30**, 434-440.

Lukaski, H.C., Johnson, P.E., Bolonchuk, W.W., & Lykken, G.I. (1985). Assessment of fat-free mass using bioelectric impedance measurements of the human body. *American Journal of Clinical Nutrition*, **41**, 810-817.

Malina, R.M. (1973). Comparative studies of blacks and whites in the United States. In K.S. Miller and R.M. Dreger (Eds.), *Biological Substrata* (pp. 53-123). New York: Seminar Press.

Martin, A.D., Drinkwater, D.T., & Clarys, J.P. (1992). Effects of skin thickness and skinfold compressibility on skinfold thickness measurements. *American Journal of Human Biology*, **4**, 453-460.

Martorell, R., Mendoza, F., Mueller, W.H., & Pawson, I.G. (1988). Which side to measure: Right or left? In T.G. Lohman, A.F. Roche, & R. Martorell (Eds.), *Anthropometric standardization reference manual* (pp. 87-91). Champaign, IL: Human Kinetics.

Mayhew, J.L., Piper, F.C., Koss, M.A., & Montaldi, D.H. (1983). Prediction of body composition in female athletes. *Journal of Sports Medicine*, **23**, 333-340.

Mazess, R.B. (1991). Do bioimpedance changes reflect weight, not composition? *American Journal of Clinical Nutrition*, **53**, 178-179. (Letter to editor)

Mazess, R.B., Barden, H.S., Bisek, J.P., & Hanson, J. (1990). Dual-energy x-ray absorptiometry for total-body and regional bone-mineral and soft-tissue composition. *American Journal of Clinical Nutrition*, **51**, 1106-1112.

Mazess, R.B., Barden, H.S., & Ohlrich, E.S. (1990). Skeletal and body-composition effects of anorexia nervosa. *American Journal of Clinical Nutrition*, **52**, 438-441.

McHugh, D., Baumgartner, R.N., Stauber, P.M., Wayne, S., Hicks, V.L. & Heyward, V.H. (1993). Bone mineral in Native American women from New Mexico. In K.J. Ellis, & J.D. Eastman (Eds.), *Human body composition: In vivo methods, models and assessment* (pp. 87-88). New York: Plenum.

McLean, K.P., & Skinner, J.S. (1992). Validity of Futrex-5000 for body composition determination. *Medicine and Science in Sports and Exercise*, **24**, 253-258.

Micozzi, M.S., Albanes, D., Jones, Y., & Chumlea, W.C. (1986). Correlations of body mass indices with weight, stature, and body composition in men and women in NHANES I and II. *American Journal of Clinical Nutrition*, **44**, 725-731.

Mitchell, C.O., Rose, J., Familoni, B., Winters, S., & Ling, F. (1993). The use of multifrequency bioelectrical impedance analysis to estimate fluid volume changes as a function of the menstrual cycle. In K.J. Ellis & J.D. Eastman (Eds.), *Human body composition: In vivo methods, models and assessment* (pp. 189-191). New York: Plenum.

Morrow, J.R., Fridye, T., & Monaghen, S.D. (1986). Generalizability of the AAHPERD health-related skinfold test. *Research Quarterly for Exercise and Sport*, **57**, 187-195.

Morrow, J.R., Jackson, A.S., Bradley, P.W., & Hartung, G.H. (1986). Accuracy of measured and predicted residual lung volume on body density measurement. *Medicine and Science in Sports and Exercise*, **18**, 647-652.

Mueller, W.H., Shoup, R.F., & Malina, R.M. (1982). Fat patterning in athletes in relation to ethnic origin and sport. *Annals of Human Biology*, **9**, 371-376.

Nagamine, S., & Suzuki, S. (1964). Anthropometry and body composition of Japanese young men and women. *Human Biology*, **36**, 8-15.

Nakadomo, F., Tanaka, K., Hazama, T., & Maeda K. (1990). Validation of body composition assessed by bioelectrical impedance analysis. *Japanese Journal of Applied Physiology*, **20**, 321-330.

National Institutes of Health. (1985). Health implications of obesity: National Institutes of Health consensus development statement. *Annals of Internal Medicine, 103,* 1073-1077.

National Research Council. (1989). *Diet and health. Implications for reducing chronic disease risk.* Washington, DC: National Academy Press.

Nattiv, A., Agostina, R., Drinkwater, B., & Yeager, K. (1993). The female athlete triad. *Clinics in Sports Medicine, 13,* 405-418.

Nelson, D.A., Feingold, M., Bolin, F. & Parfitt, A.M. (1991). Principal components analysis of regional bone density in black and white women: Relationship to body size and composition. *American Journal of Physical Anthropology, 86,* 507-514.

Nielsen, D.H., Cassady, S.L., Janz, K.F., Cook, J.S., Hansen, J.R., & Wu, Y. (1993). Criterion methods of body composition analysis for children and adolescents. *American Journal of Human Biology, 5,* 211-223.

Nielsen, D.H., Cassady, S.L., Wacker, L.M., Wessels, A.K., Wheelock, B.J., & Oppliger, R.A. (1992). Validation of the Futrex-5000 near-infrared spectrophotometer analyzer for assessment of body composition. *Journal of Orthopaedic and Sports Physical Therapy, 16,* 281-287.

Nilsson, B.E., & Westlin, N.E. (1971). Bone density in athletes. *Clincial Orthopaedics, 77,* 179-182.

Norris, K.H. (1983). Instrumental techniques for measuring quality of agricultural crops. In M. Lieberman (Ed.), *Post-harvest physiology and crop preservation* (pp. 471-484). New York: Plenum.

Oppliger, R.A., Nielsen, D.H., Hoegh, J.E., & Vance, C.G. (1991). Bioelectrical impedance prediction of fat-free mass for high school wrestlers validated. *Medicine and Science in Sports and Exercise, 23,* S73. (Abstract)

Oppliger, R.A., Nielsen, D.H., Shetler, A.C., Crowley, E.T., & Albright, J.P. (1992). Body composition of collegiate football players: Bioelectrical impedance and skinfolds compared to hydrostatic weighing. *Journal of Orthopaedic and Sports Physical Therapy, 15,* 187-192.

Oppliger, R.A., Nielsen, D.H., & Vance, C.G. (1991). Wrestlers' minimal weight: Anthropometry, bioimpedance, and hydrostatic weighing compared. *Medicine and Science in Sports and Exercise, 23,* 247-253.

Ortiz, O., Russell, M., Daley, T.L., Baumgartner, R.N., Waki, M., Lichtman, S., Wang, J., Pierson, R.N., & Heymsfield, S.B. (1992). Differences in skeletal muscle and bone mineral mass between black and white females and their relevance to estimates of body composition. *American Journal of Clinical Nutrition, 55,* 8-13.

Paijmans, I.J.M., Wilmore, K.M., & Wilmore, J.H. (1992). Use of skinfolds and bioelectrical impedance for body composition assessment after weight reduction. *Journal of the American College of Nutrition, 11,* 145-151.

Pavlou, K.N., Steffee, W.P., Lerman, R.H., & Burrows, B.A. (1985). Effects of dieting and exercise on lean body mass, oxygen uptake, and strength. *Medicine and Science in Sports and Exercise, 17,* 466-471.

Pawson, I.G., Martorell, R., & Mendoza, F.E. (1991). Prevalence of overweight and obesity in US Hispanic populations. *American Journal of Clinical Nutrition, 53,* 1522S-1528S.

Pedhazuer, E.J. (1982). *Multiple regression in behavioral research.* New York: CBS College.

Peters, D., Fox, K., Armstrong, N., Sharpe, P., & Bell, M. (1992). Assessment of children's abdominal fat distribution by magnetic resonance imaging and anthropometry. *International Journal of Obesity, 16* (Suppl. 2), S35. (Abstract)

Pierson, R.N., Wang, J., Heymsfield, S.B., Russell-Aulet, M., Mazariegos, M., Tierney, M., Smith, R., Thornton, J.C., Kehayias, J., Weber, D.A., & Dilmanian, F.A. (1991). Measuring body fat: Calibrating the rulers. Intermethod comparisons in 389 normal Caucasian subjects. *American Journal of Physiology*, **261**, E103-E108.

Pollock, M.L., & Jackson, A.S.(1984). Research progress in validation of clincal methods of assessing body composition. *Medicine and Science in Sports and Exercise*, **16**, 606-613.

Pollock, M.L., Schmidt, D.H., & Jackson, A.S. (1980). Measurement of cardiorespiratory fitness and body composition in the clinical setting. *Comprehensive Therapy*, **6**, 12-27.

Quatrochi, J.A., Hicks, V.L., Heyward, V.H., Colville, B.C., Cook, K.L., Jenkins, K.A., & Wilson, W. (1992). Relationship of optical density and skinfold measurements: Effects of age and level of body fatness. *Research Quarterly for Exercise and Sports*, **63**, 402-409.

Rabeneck, L., Risser, J.M., Crane, M.M., McCabe, B.K., & Worsley, J.B. (1993). A comparison of anthropometry and bioelectrical impedance in the estimation of body composition in HIV-infected individuals. *Nutrition Research*, **13**, 275-285.

Rising, R., Swinburn, B., Larson, K., & Ravussin, E. (1991). Body composition in Pima Indians: Validation of bioelectrical resistance. *American Journal of Clinical Nutrition*, **53**, 594-598.

Roby, F.B., Kempema, J.M., Lohman, T.G., Williams, D.P., & Tipton, C.M. (1991). Can the same equation be used to predict minimal wrestling weight in Hispanic and Non-Hispanic wrestlers? *Medicine and Science in Sports and Exercise*, **23**, S29. (Abstract)

Ross, R., Leger, L., Marliss, E.B., Morris, D.V., & Gougeon, R. (1991). Adipose tissue distribution changes during rapid weight loss in obese adults. *International Journal of Obesity*, **15**, 733-739.

Ross, R., Leger, L., Martin, P., & Roy, R. (1989). Sensitivity of bioelectrical impedance to detect changes in human body composition. *Journal of Applied Physiology*, **67**, 1643-1648.

Roubenoff, R., Kehayias, J.J., Dawson-Hughes, B., & Heymsfield, S.B. (1993). Use of dual-energy x-ray absorptiometry in body-composition studies: Not yet a "gold standard." *American Journal of Clinical Nutrition*, **58**, 589-591.

Samet, J.M., Coultas, D.B., Howard, C.A., Skipper, B.J., & Hanis, C.L. (1988). Diabetes, gallbladder disease, obesity, and hypertension among Hispanics in New Mexico. *American Journal of Epidemiology*, **128**, 1302-1311.

Sanborn, C.F. (1986). Etiology of athletic amenorrhea. In J.L.Puhl, & C.H. Brown (Eds.), *The menstrual cycle and physical activity* (pp. 45-58). Champaign, IL: Human Kinetics.

Sanborn, C.F., & Wagner, W.W. (1987). Response to Nelson and Evans. *Medicine and Science in Sports and Exercise*, **19**, 621-622.

Sawai, Mutoh, & Miyashita (1990). *Study on effectiveness, when applied to Japanese Natives, of an instrument for measurement of body fat with near-infrared interactance technology.* Translated and reprinted from the annals of Tokyo University by Futrex, Inc.

Saxenhofer, H., Scheidegger, J., Descoeudres, C., Jaeger, P., & Horber, F.F. (1992). Impact of dialysis modality on body composition in patients with end-stage renal disease. *Clinical Nephrology*, **38**, 219-223.

Scherf, J., Franklin, B.A., Lucas, C.P., Stevenson, D., & Rubenfire, M. (1986). Validity of skinfold thickness measures of formerly obese adults. *American Journal of Clincial Nutrition, 43*, 128-135.

Schoeller, D.A., & Kushner, R.F. (1991). Reply to R.B. Mazess and P. Deurenberg et al. *American Journal of Clinical Nutrition, 53*, 180. (Letter to editor)

Schols, A.M., Wouters, E.F., Soeters, P.B., & Westerterp, K.R. (1991). Body composition by bioelectrical-impedance analysis compared with deuterium dilution and skinfold anthropometry in patients with chronic pulmonary disease. *American Journal of Clinical Nutrition, 53*, 421-424.

Schutte, J.E., Townsend, E.J., Hugg, J., Shoup, R.F., Malina, R.M., & Blomqvist, C.G. (1984). Denisty of lean body mass is greater in blacks than in whites. *Journal of Applied Physiology, 56*, 1647-1649.

Segal, K.R., Burastero, S., Chun, A., Coronel, P., Pierson, R.N., & Wang, J. (1991). Estimation of extracellular and total body water by multiple-frequency bioelectrical-impedance measurement. *American Journal of Clinical Nutrition, 54*, 26-29.

Segal, K.R., Gutin, B., Presta, E., Wang, J., & Van Itallie, T.B. (1985). Estimation of human body composition by electrical impedance methods: A comparative study. *Journal of Applied Physiology, 58*, 1565-1571.

Segal, K.R., Kral, J.G., Wang, J., Pierson, R.N., & Van Itallie, T.B. (1987). Estimation of body water distribution by bioelectrical impedance. *Federation Proceedings, 46*, 1334. (Abstract)

Segal, K.R., Van Loan, M., Fitzgerald, P.I., Hodgdon, J.A., & Van Itallie, T.B. (1988). Lean body mass estimation by bioelectrical impedance analysis: A four-site cross-validation study. *American Journal of Clinical Nutrition, 47*, 7-14.

Segal, K.R., Wang, J., Gutin, B., Pierson, R.N., & Van Itallie, T.B. (1987). Hydration and potassium content of lean body mass: Effects of body fat, sex, and age. *American Journal of Clinical Nutrition, 45*, 865. (Abstract)

Seidell, J.C., Bjorntorp, P., Sjostrom, L., Sannerstedt, R., Krotkiewski, M., & Kvist, H. (1989). Regional distribution of muscle and fat mass in men--New insight into the risk of abdominal obesity using computed tomography. *International Journal of Obesity, 13*, 289-303.

Seidell, J.C., Oosterlee, A., Thijssen, M., Burema, J., Deurenberg, P., Hautvast, J., & Ruijs, J. (1987). Assessment of intra-abdominal and subcutaneous abdominal fat: Relation between anthropometry and computed tomography. *American Journal of Clinical Nutrition, 45*, 7-13.

Seip, R., & Weltman, A. (1991). Validity of skinfold and girth based regression equations for the prediction of body composition in obese adults. *American Journal of Human Biology, 3*, 91-95.

Selinger, A. (1977). *The body as a three component system.* Unpublished doctoral dissertation, University of Illinois, Urbana.

Sinning, W.E., Dolny, D.G., Little, K.D., Cunningham, L.N., Racaniello, A., Siconolfi, S.F., & Sholes, J.L. (1985). Validity of "generalized" equations for body composition analysis in male athletes. *Medicine and Science in Sports and Exercise, 17*, 124-130.

Sinning, W.E., & Wilson, J.R. (1984). Validity of "generalized" equations for body composition analysis in women athletes. *Research Quarterly for Exercise and Sport, 55*, 153-160.

Siri, W.E. (1961). Body composition from fluid spaces and density: Analysis of methods. In J. Brozek & A. Henschel (Eds.), *Techniques for measuring body composition* (pp. 223-244). Washington, DC: National Academy of Sciences.

Slaughter, M.H., Lohman, T.G., Boileau, R.A., Horswill, C.A., Stillman, R.J., Van Loan, M.D., & Bemben, D.A. (1988). Skinfold equations for estimation of body fatness in children and youth. *Human Biology*, **60**, 709-723.

Slavin, J.L. (1988). Eating disorders in women athletes. In J. Puhl, C.H. Brown, & R. Voy (Eds.), *Sport science perspectives for women* (pp. 189-198). Champaign, IL: Human Kinetics.

Sloan A.W. (1967). Estimation of body fat in young men. *Journal of Applied Physiology*, **23**, 311-315.

Sloan, A.W., Burt, J.J., & Blyth, C.S. (1962). Estimation of body fat in young women. *Journal of Applied Physiology*, **17**, 967-970.

Smalley, K.J., Knerr, A.N., Kendrick, Z.V., Colliver, J.A., & Owens, O.E. (1990). Reassessment of body mass indices. *American Journal of Clinical Nutrition*, **52**, 405-408.

Smith, D.M., Khairi, M.R.A., Norton, J., & Johnston, C.C. (1976). Age and activity effects on the rate of bone mineral loss. *Journal of Clinical Investigation*, **58**, 716-721.

Snow-Harter, C.M. (1993). Bone health and prevention of osteoporosis in active and athletic women. *Clinics in Sports Medicine*, **13**, 389-404.

Sparling, P.B., Millard-Stafford, M.L., Rosskopf, L.B., DiCarlo, L.J., & Hinson, B.T. (1993). Body composition by bioelectric impedance and densitometry in black women. *American Journal of Human Biology*, **5**, 111-117.

Spicher, V., Roulet, M., Schaffner, C., & Schutz, Y. (1993). Bio-electrical impedance analysis for estimation of fat-free mass and muscle mass in cystic fibrosis patients. *European Journal of Pediatrics*, **152**, 222-225.

Steen, S.N., & Brownell, K.D. (1990). Patterns of weight loss and regain in wrestlers: Has the tradition changed? *Medicine and Science in Sports and Exercise*, **6**, 762-768.

Stevens, J., Keil, J.E., Rust, P.F., Tyroler, H.A., Davis, C.E., & Gazes, P.C. (1992). Body mass index and body girth as predictors of mortality in black and white women. *Archives of Internal Medicine*, **152**, 1257-1262.

Stokes, T.M., Sinning, W.E., Morgan, A.L., & Ellison, J.D. (1993). Bioimpedance (BI) estimation of fat free mass in black and white women. *Medicine and Science in Sports and Exercise*, **25**, S162. (Abstract)

Stolarczyk, L.M., Heyward, V., Goodman, J., Grant, J., Kessler, K., Kocina, P., Wilmerding, V. (1995). Predictive accuracy of bioelectrical impedance in estimating fat-free mass of Hispanic women. *Medicine and Science in Sports and Exercise*.

Stolarczyk, L.M., Heyward, V.H., Hicks, V.L., & Baumgartner, R.N. (1994). Predictive accuracy of bioelectrical impedance in estimating body composition of Native American women. *American Journal of Clinical Nutrition*, **59**, 964-970.

Strain, G.W., & Zumoff, B. (1992). The relationship of weight-height indices of obesity to body fat content. *Journal of the American College of Nutrition*, **11**, 715-718.

Sugimoto, T., Tsutsumi, M., Fujii, Y., Kawakatsu, M., Negishi, H., Lee, M.C., Tsai, K., Fukase, M., & Fujita, T. (1992). Comparison of bone mineral content among Japanese, Koreans, and Taiwanese assessed by dual-photon absorptiometry. *Journal of Bone and Mineral Research*, **7**, 153-159.

Svendsen, O.L., Haarbo, J., Heitmann, B.L., Gotfredsen, A., & Christiansen, C. (1991). Measurement of body fat in elderly subjects by dual-energy x-ray absorptiometry, bioelectrical impedance, and anthropometry. *American Journal of Clinical Nutrition*, **53**, 1117-1123.

Svendsen, O.L., Hassager, C., Bergmann, I., & Christiansen, C. (1992). Measurement of abdominal and intra-abdominal fat in postmenopausal women by dual energy x-ray absorptiometry and anthropometry: Comparison with computerized tomography. *International Journal of Obesity, 17*, 45-51.

Tanaka, K., Hiyama, T., Watanabe, Y., Asano, K., Takeda, M., Hayakawa, Y., & Nakadomo, F. (1993). Assessment of exercise-induced alterations in body composition of patients with coronary heart disease. *European Journal of Applied Physiology, 66*, 321-327.

Tanaka, K., Nakadomo, F., Watanabe, K., Inagaki, A., Kim, H.K., & Matsuura, Y. (1992). Body composition prediction equations based on bioelectrical impedance and anthropometric variables for Japanese obese women. *American Journal of Human Biology, 4*, 739-745.

Teran, J.C., Sparks, K.E., Quinn, L.M., Fernandez, B.S., Krey, S.H., & Steffee, W.P. (1991). Percent body fat in obese white females predicted by anthropometric measurements. *American Journal of Clinical Nutrition, 53*, 7-13.

Thomas, D.Q., & Whitehead, J.R. (1993). Body composition assessment: Some practical answers to teachers' questions. *Journal of Physical Education, Recreation, and Dance, 63*, 16-19.

Thomasett, A. (1962). Bio-electrical properties of tissue impedance measurements. *Lyon Medical, 207*, 107-118.

Thorland, W.G., Johnson, G.O., Cisar, C.J., & Housh, T.J. (1987). Estimation of minimal wrestling weight using measures of body build and body composition. *International Journal of Sports Medicine, 8*, 365-370.

Thorland, W.G., Johnson, G.O., Tharp, G.D., Fagot, T.G., & Hammer, R.W. (1984). Validity of anthropometric equations for the estimation of body density in adolescent athletes. *Medicine and Science in Sports and Exercise, 16*, 77-81.

Thorland, W.G., Tipton, C.M., Lohman, T.G., Bowers, R.W., Housh, T.J., Johnson, G.O., Kelly, J.M., Oppliger, R.A., & Tcheng, T. (1991). Midwest wrestling study: Prediction of minimal weight for high school wrestlers. *Medicine and Science in Sports and Exercise, 23*, 1102-1110.

Tipton, C.M., & Oppliger, R.A. (1984). The Iowa wrestling study: Lessons for physicians. *Iowa Medicine, 74*, 381-385.

Tran, Z.V., & Weltman, A. (1988). Predicting body composition of men from girth measurements. *Human Biology, 60*, 167-175.

Tran, Z.V., & Weltman, A. (1989). Generalized equation for predicting body density of women from girth measurements. *Medicine and Science in Sports and Exercise, 21*, 101-104.

Tsai, K.S., Huang, K.M., Chieng, P.U., & Cheng, C.T., (1991). Bone mineral density of normal Chinese women in Taiwan. *Calcified Tissue Research, 48*, 161-166.

Tsunenari, T., Tsutsumi, M., Ohno, K., Yamamoto, Y., Kawakatsu, M., Shimogaki, K., Negishi, H., Sugimoto, T., Fukase, M., & Fujita, T. (1993). Age- and gender-related changes in body composition in Japanese subjects. *Journal of Bone and Mineral Research, 8*, 397-402.

U.S. Department of Commerce. (1991, June 12). Census Bureau Releases 1990 census counts on specific racial groups. *United States Department of Commerce News, CB91*, 215.

U.S. Department of Health and Human Services. (1988). *The Surgeon General's report on nutrition and health* (DHHS [PHS] Publication No. 88-50210). Washington, DC: U.S. Government Printing Office.

U.S. Department of Health and Human Services. (1990). *Healthy people 2000: National health promotion and disease prevention objectives* (DHHS [PHS] Publication No. 90-50212). Washington, D.C., U.S. Government Printing Office.

Vague, J. (1947). La differenciation sexuelle facteur determinant des formes de l'obesite. *La Presse Medicale*, **30**, 339-340.

Vaisman, N., Corey, M., Rossi, M.F., Goldberg, E., & Pencharz, P. (1988). Changes in body composition during refeeding of patients with anorexia nervosa. *Journal of Pediatrics*, **113**, 925-929.

Vaisman, N., Rossi, M.F., Goldberg, E., Dibden, L.J., Wykes, L.J., & Pencharz, P.B. (1988). Energy expenditure and body composition in patients with anorexia nervosa. *Journal of Pediatrics*, **113**, 919-924.

Valdez, R. (1991). A simple model-based index of abdominal adiposity. *Journal of Clinical Epidemiology*, **44**, 955-956.

Valdez, R., Seidell, J.C., Ahn, Y.I., & Weiss, K.M. (1992). A new index of abdominal adiposity as an indicator of risk for cardiovascular disease. A cross-population study. *International Journal of Obesity*, **17**, 77-82.

van der Kooy, K., Leenen, R., Deurenberg, P., Seidell, J.C., Westerterp, K.R., & Hautvast, J.G. (1992). Changes in fat-free mass in obese subjects after weight loss: A comparison of body composition measures. *International Journal of Obesity*, **16**, 675-683.

van der Kooy, K., Leenen, R., Seidell, J.C., Deurenberg, P., Droop, A., & Bakker, C.J.G. (1993). Waist-hip ratio is a poor predictor of changes in visceral fat. *American Journal of Clinical Nutrition*, **57**, 327-333.

Van Loan, M.D. (1990). Bioelectrical impedance analysis to determine fat-free mass, total body water and body fat. *Sports Medicine*, **10**, 205-217.

Van Loan, M.D. Boileau, R.A., Christ, C.B., Elmore, B., Lohman, T.G., Going, S.B., & Carswell, C. (1990). Association of bioelectric resistance impedance with fat-free mass and total body water estimates of body composition. *American Journal of Human Biology*, **2**, 219-226.

Van Loan, M.D., & Mayclin, P.L. (1987). Bioelectrical impedance analysis: Is it a a reliable estimator of lean body mass and total body water? *Human Biology*, **59**, 299-309.

Van Loan, M.D., & Mayclin, P.L. (1992). Body composition assessment: Dual-energy x-ray absorptiometry (DEXA) compared to reference methods. *European Journal of Clinical Nutrition*, **46**, 125-130.

Van Loan, M.D., Withers, P., Matthie, J., & Mayclin, P.L. (1993). Use of bio-impedance spectroscopy (BIS) to determine extracellular fluid (ECF), intracellular fluid (ICF), total body water (TBW), and fat-free mass (FFM). In K.J. Ellis, & J.D. Eastman (Eds.), *Human body composition: In vivo methods, models and assessment* (pp. 67-70). New York: Plenum.

Vazquez, J.A., & Janosky, J.E. (1991). Validity of bioelectrical-impedance analysis in measuring changes in lean body mass during weight reduction. *American Journal of Clinical Nutrition*, **54**, 970-975.

Vickery, M.C., Cureton, K.J., & Collins, M.A. (1988). Prediction of body density from skinfolds in black and white young men. *Human Biology*, **60**, 135-149.

Waki, M., Kral, J.G., Mazariegos, M., Wang, J., Pierson, R.N., & Heymsfield, S.B. (1991). Relative expansion of extracellular fluid in obese vs. nonobese women. *American Journal of Physiology*, **261**, E199-E203.

Wang, J., Heymsfield, S.B., Aulet, M., Thornton, J.C., & Pierson, R.N. (1989). Body fat from body density: Underwater weighing vs. dual-photon absorptiometry. *American Journal of Physiology*, **256**, E829-E834.

Wang, J., Thornton, J.C., Burastero, S., Heymsfield, S.B., & Pierson, R.N. (1995). Bio-impedance analysis for estimation of total body potassium, total body water, and fat-free mass in white, black, and Asian adults. *American Journal of Human Biology*, **7**, 33-40.

Wang, J., Thornton, J.C., Russell, M., Burastero, S., Heymsfield, S., & Pierson, R.N. (1994). Asians have lower body mass index (BMI) but higher percent body fat than do whites: Comparison of anthropometric measurements. *American Journal of Clinical Nutrition*, **60**, 23-28.

Watanabe, K., Nakadomo, F., Tanaka, K., Kim, K., & Maeda, K.(1993). Estimation of fat-free mass from bioelectrical impedance and anthropometric variables in Japanese girls. *Medicine and Science in Sports and Exercise*, **25**, S163. (Abstract)

Weits, T., Van der Beek, E.J., Wedel, M. & Ter Haar Romeny, B.M. (1988). Computed tomography measurement of abdominal fat deposition in relation to anthropometry. *International Journal of Obesity*, **12**, 217-225.

Weltman, A., Levine, S., Seip, R.L., & Tran, Z.V. (1988). Accurate assessment of body composition in obese females. *American Journal of Clinical Nutrition*, **48**, 1179-1183.

Weltman, A., Seip, R.L., & Tran, Z.V. (1987). Practical assessment of body composition in adult obese males. *Human Biology*, **59**, 523-535.

Welty, T.K. (1991). Health implications of obesity in American Indians and Alaska Natives. *American Journal of Clinical Nutrition*, **53**, 1616S-1620S.

White, F., Periera, L., & Garner, J.B. (1986). Associations of body mass index and waist-hip ratio with hypertension. *Canadian Medical Association Journal*, **135**, 313-320.

Williams, D.P., Going, S.B., Lohman, T.G., Harsha, D.W., Srinivasan, S.R., Webber, L.S., & Berenson, G.S. (1992). Body fatness and risk for elevated blood pressure, total cholesterol, and serum lipoprotein ratios in children and adolescents. *American Journal of Public Health*, **82**, 358-363.

Williams, D.P., Going, S.B., Lohman, T.G., Hewitt, M.J., & Haber, A.E. (1992). Estimation of body fat from skinfold thicknesses in middle-aged and older men and women: A multiple component approach. *American Journal of Human Biology*, **4**, 595-605.

Williams, D.P., Going, S.B., Massett, M.P., Lohman, T.G., Bare, L.A., & Hewitt, M.J. (1993). Aqueous and mineral fractions of the fat-free body and their relation to body fat estimates in men and women aged 49-82 years. In K.J. Ellis, & J.D. Eastman (Eds.), *Human body composition: In vivo methods, models and assessment* (pp. 109-113). New York: Plenum.

Williamson, D.F., Kahn, H.S., & Byers, T. (1991). The 10-y incidence of obesity and major weight gain in black and white US women aged 30-55 y. *American Journal of Clinical Nutrition*, **53**, 1515S-1518S.

Wilmore, J.H. (1983). Body composition in sport and exercise: Directions for future research. *Medicine and Science in Sports and Exercise*, **15**, 21-31.

Wilmore, J.H., & Behnke, A.R. (1969). An anthropometric estimation of body density and lean body weight in young men. *Journal of Applied Physiology*, **27**, 25-31.

Wilmore, J.H., & Behnke, A.R. (1970). An anthropometric estimation of body density and lean body weight in young women. *American Journal of Clinical Nutrition*, **23**, 267-274.

Wilmore, J.H., Frisancho, R.A., Gordon, C.C., Himes, J.H., Martin, A.D., Martorell, R., & Seefeldt, V.D. (1988). Body breadth equipment and measurement techniques. In T.G. Lohman, A.F. Roche, & R. Martorell (Eds.), *Anthropometric standardization reference manual* (pp. 27-38). Champaign, IL: Human Kinetics.

Wilmore, K.M., McBride, P.J., & Wilmore, J.H. (1994). Comparison of bioelectric impedance and near-infrared interactance for human body composition assessment in a population of self-perceived overweight adults. *International Journal of Obesity*, **18**, 375-381.

Wilson, W.L., & Heyward, V.H. (1993a). Effects of skintone, skinfold, and mid-arm muscle area on optical density measurements at the biceps site. *Medicine and Science in Sports and Exercise*, **25**, S60. (Abstract)

Wilson, W.L., & Heyward, V.H. (1993b). Validation of the near-infrared interactance method for black, Hispanic, Native American and white men, 20 to 50 years. In K.J. Ellis, & J.D. Eastman (Eds.), *Human body composition: In vivo methods, models and assessment* (pp. 389-392). New York: Plenum.

Wilson, W.L., Heyward, V.H., Cook, K.L., Hicks, V.L., Jenkins, K.A., Quatrochi, J.A., & Colville, B.C. (1992). Predictive accuracy of bioelectrical impedance equations corrected for fat-free body size. *American Journal of Human Biology*, **4**, 319-326.

Withers, R.T., Craig, N.P, Bourdon, P.C., & Norton, K.I. (1987). Relative body fat and anthropometric prediction of body density of male athletes. *European Journal of Applied Physiology*, **56**, 191-200.

Withers, R.T., Whittingham, N.O., Norton, K.I., La Forgia, J., Ellis, M.W., & Crockett, A. (1987). Relative body fat and anthropometric prediction of body density of female athletes. *European Journal of Applied Physiology*, **56**, 169-180.

World Health Organization. (1988). *Measuring obesity-classification and description of anthropometric data*. Report of a WHO Regional Office Consultation on the Epidemiology of Obesity. Copenhagen, Denmark: WHO Regional Office for Europe, Nutrition Unit. (Document EUR/ICP/NUT 125)

Yeager, K.K., Agostini, R., Nattiv, A., & Drinkwater, B. (1993). The female athlete triad: Disordered eating, amenorrhea, osteoporosis. *Medicine and Science in Sports and Exercise*, **25**, 775-777.

Zamboni, M., Armellini, F., Milani, M.P., De Marchi, M., Todesco, T., Robbi, R., Bergamo-Andreis, I.V., & Bosello, O. (1992). Body fat distribution in pre- and post-menopausal women: Metabolic and anthropometric variables and their interrelationships. *International Journal of Obesity*, **16**, 495-504.

Zando, K.A., & Robertson, R.J. (1987). The validity and reliability of the Cramer Skyndex caliper in the estimation of percent body fat. *Athletic Training*, **22**, 23-25, 79.

Zillikens, M.C. & Conway, J.M. (1990). Anthropometry in blacks: Applicability of generalized skinfold equations and differences in fat patterning between blacks and whites. *American Journal of Clinical Nutrition*, **52**, 45-51.

Zillikens, M.C., & Conway, J.M. (1991). Estimation of total body water by bioelectrical impedance analysis in blacks. *American Journal of Human Biology*, **3**, 25-32.

Zillikens, M.C., van den Berg, J.W., Wilson, J.H., Rietveld, T., & Swart, G.R. (1992). The validity of bioelectrical impedance analysis in estimating body water in patients with cirrhosis. *Journal of Hepatology*, **16**, 59-65.

Index

About the Authors

Dr. Vivian H. Heyward, a professor of exercise science at the University of New Mexico (UNM) for 21 years, brings a wealth of knowledge and experience to this book.

Dr. Heyward's interest in body composition was first stimulated by her personal experience with competitive bodybuilding. She also studied and worked with Drs. Tim Lohman and Scott Going, body composition specialists at the University of Arizona. The experience of teaching body composition courses at UNM allowed Dr. Heyward to identify and bridge the gap between body composition research and practice.

Dr. Heyward's research dealing with body composition assessment in a variety of population groups has appeared in such prestigious journals as the *American Journal of Clinical Nutrition, American Journal of Human Biology,* and *International Journal of Sports Nutrition.* She also conducts numerous body composition workshops for nutritionists, health and fitness professionals, physical therapists, and nurses.

Dr. Heyward is certified by the American College of Sports Medicine (ACSM) as a health and fitness instructor, and she is a former chair of the Exercise Physiology Academy of the National Association for Sport and Physical Education and a member of the ACSM and the American Society of Clinical Nutrition.

Lisa M. Stolarczyk received her PhD in exercise science from the University of New Mexico. She has both research and clinical experience with body composition assessment.

As a research assistant at the Center for Exercise Body Composition Laboratory at UNM, Dr. Stolarczyk gained invaluable knowledge about body composition field methods and equations for measuring body fat of clients. Her research has been published in many journals including the *American Journal of Clinical Nutrition,* the *Journal of Strength and Conditioning Research,* and *Medicine and Science in Sports and Exercise.*

Dr. Stolarczyk has taught Advanced Meatabolism at the University of Zulia in Maracaibo, Venezuela, and Test and Measurements at UNM. She is a member of ACSM and has presented research papers at the organization's regional and national meetings.

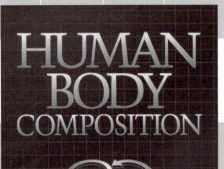